REDUCE
CHILD
OBESITY

A GUIDE FOR USING
THE KID'S CHOICE PROGRAM
IN SCHOOL AND AT HOME

HELEN HENDY, KEITH WILLIAMS,
AND THOMAS CAMISE

ROWMAN & LITTLEFIELD EDUCATION
A DIVISION OF
ROWMAN & LITTLEFIELD
Lanham • Boulder • New York • Toronto • Plymouth, UK

Published by Rowman & Littlefield Education
A division of Rowman & Littlefield
4501 Forbes Boulevard, Suite 200, Lanham, Maryland 20706
www.rowman.com

10 Thornbury Road, Plymouth PL6 7PP, United Kingdom

British Library Cataloguing in Publication Information Available

Library of Congress Cataloging-in-Publication Data

Hendy, Helen.
  Reduce child obesity : a guide for using the kid's choice program in school and at home / Helen Hendy, Keith Williams, and Thomas Camise.
  pages cm
  Includes bibliographical references.
    ISBN 978-1-61048-792-4 (pbk. :alk. paper) — ISBN 978-1-61048-793-1 (electronic) 1. Obesity in children—Prevention. 2. Obesity in children—Diet therapy. 3. Weight loss. I. Title.
  RJ399.C6H46 2013
  618.92'398--dc23   2013027166

∞™ The paper used in this publication meets the minimum requirements of American National Standard for Information Sciences—Permanence of Paper for Printed Library Materials, ANSI/NISO Z39.48-1992.
Printed in the United States of America

DEDICATION

To our families

CONTENTS

LIST OF CHAPTER INSERTS

Chapter 8

Chapter 9

1

INTRODUCTION TO THE KID'S CHOICE PROGRAM

THE PROBLEM OF OVERWEIGHT CHILDREN

Over 30% of American schoolchildren are now overweight or obese (Cole et al., 2000; Wang & Beydown, 2007) and they face a number of health problems including diabetes, high blood pressure, gallstones, sleep apnea, and orthopedic abnormalities such as bowed legs and back problems (Must & Strauss, 1999). Social problems associated with child overweight include peer teasing and being stereotyped as lazy, stupid, ugly, and worthless (Davison & Birch, 2001; Latner & Stunkard, 2003; Turnbull et al., 2000). Psychological problems include poor body image, low self-esteem, depression, anxiety disorders, and self-rated quality of life as low as that of children with cancer (Schwimmer et al., 2003; Williams et al., 2001). Unfortunately, children's unhealthy eating habits are rarely just a "phase" and they continue into adulthood (Mikkila et al., 2004).

American children live in a "supersize me" environment with snack foods and fast-food restaurants offering many high-fat and high-sugar items in large portions (Deckelbaum & Williams, 2001; Rozin et al., 2006). Children are repeatedly exposed to media advertisements for these foods (Harris et al., 2009; Lobstein & Dibb, 2005), with increasing numbers of children skipping breakfast, drinking soda rather than milk, and rarely eating fruits and vegetables (FV) (Jahns et al., 2001; Jones et al., 2010; Ludwig et al., 2001). Children also spend increasing amounts of time in sedentary activities such as watching television, using a computer, and playing videogames (Brown et al., 2011; Mendoza et al., 2007). (Please see Textbox 1.1 for suggested readings on child obesity.)

THE PROBLEM OF PICKY EATING

Up to 50% of children in the United States are "picky eaters" who accept only a limited variety of foods (Bryant-Waugh et al., in press). Often, picky eaters completely reject fruits, vegetables, and regular-

---

TEXTBOX 1.1 READINGS ON CHILD OBESITY

Centers for Disease Control and Prevention. (2000). *School health index for physical activity and health eating: A self-assessment and planning guide.* Atlanta, GA: author.

Cole, T. J., Bellizzi, M. C., Flegal, K. M., & Dietz, W. H. (2000). Establishing a standard definition for child overweight and obesity world-wide: International survey. *British Medical Journal, 320,* 1–6.

Latner, J. D., & Stunkard, A. J. (2003). Getting worse: The stigmatization of obese children. *Obesity Research, 11,* 452–456.

Must, A., & Strauss, R. S. (1999). Risks and consequences of childhood and adolescent obesity. *International Journal of Obesity and Related Metabolic Disorders, 23* (Suppl. 2), S2–S11.

Wang, Y., & Beydown, M. A. (2007). The obesity epidemic in the United States—Gender, age, socioeconomic, racial/ethnic, and geographic characteristics: A systematic review and meta-regression analysis. *Epidemiological Reviews, 29,* 6–28.

Williams, C. L., Gulli, M. T., & Deckelbaum, R. J. (2001). Prevention and treatment of childhood obesity. *Current Atherosclerosis Reports, 3,* 486–497.

---

textured meats, eating instead a "beige diet" of mostly processed foods prepared with large amounts of sugar and/or fat (such as cereal, white bread, pasta, white rice, potato fries, salty chips, chocolate milk, chicken nuggets, hot dogs, and ice cream). Left untreated, picky eating may be associated with fatigue, frequent illness, slow healing, anemia, sleep difficulties, anorexia, aggression, and poor peer relationships (Falciglia et al., 2000; Marchi & Cohen, 1990; Timimi et al., 1997).

Picky eating often appears before 2 years of age and initially children may be underweight (Carruth et al., 2004; Dovey et al., 2008; Falciglia et al, 2000; Galloway et al., 2005). However, children with severe picky eating habits may also show normal weight status or even overweight (Williams et al., 2005), perhaps because of their high-fat diet, and/or because their parents give them nutritional supplements (Lockner et al., 2008; Schreck et al., 2004). Picky eaters are also exposed to media advertisements for snack foods and fast-food restaurants that encourage them to continue eating their "special meals" rather than shared family meals (Harris et al., 2009; Lobstein & Dibb, 2005; Rozin et al., 2006). (Please see Textbox 1.2 for suggested readings on picky eating.)

RECOMMENDATIONS FROM THE CDC

To avoid problems associated with children's overweight and picky eating, the Centers for Disease Control and Prevention (CDC, 2000) have recommended that children maintain a healthy weight status with a body mass index percentile score (BMI%) between 10% and 85% for their age group, with values above 85% considered at risk for overweight, and values over 95% considered obese. To determine a child's BMI% score, the body mass index is calculated (BMI = pounds/inches^2 × 704.5), then charts provided by the Centers for Disease Control and Prevention (CDC, 2000) are used to find the child's BMI% score in comparison to children of the same age and gender.

To accomplish these goals for BMI% scores and to maintain good health, the CDC has recommended that children be encouraged to learn a number of specific behaviors that include:

TEXTBOX 1.2 READINGS ON PICKY EATING

Dovey, T. M., Staples, P. A., Gibson, E. L., & Halford, J. C. G. (2008). Food neophobia and "picky/fussy" eating in children: A review. *Appetite, 50,* 181–193.

Galloway, A. T., Fiorito, L. M., Lee, Y., & Birch, L. L. (2005). Parental pressure, dietary patterns and weight status among girls who are "picky/fussy" eaters. *Journal of the American Dietetic Association, 103,* 692–698.

Hendy, H. M., Williams, K. E., Riegel, K., & Paul, C. (2010). Parent mealtime actions that mediate associations between children's fussy eating and their weight and diet. *Appetite, 54,* 191–195.

Marchi, M., & Cohen, P. (1990). Early childhood eating behaviors and adolescent eating disorders. *Journal of the American Academy of Child and Adolescent Psychiatry, 29,* 112–117.

Paul, C., Williams, K. E., Riegel, K., & Gibbons, B. (2007). Combining repeated taste exposure and escape prevention: An intervention for the treatment of extreme food selectivity. *Appetite, 49,* 708–711.

Pizzo, B., Williams, K. E., Paul, C., & Riegel, K. (2009). Jump start exit criterion: Exploring a new model of service delivery for the treatment of childhood feeding problems. *Behavioral Interventions, 24,* 195–203.

Williams, K. E., Field, D. G., & Seiverling, L. (2010). Food refusal in children: A review of the literature. *Research in Developmental Disabilities, 31,* 625–633.

Williams, K. E., Paul, C., Pizzo, B., & Riegel, K. (2008). Practice does make perfect: A longitudinal look at repeated taste exposure. *Appetite, 51,* 739–742.

- Exercise daily ("EXERCISE")
- Choose low-fat and low-sugar healthy drinks ("HDRINK")
- Eat a variety of foods, especially low-calorie, high-nutrient fruits and vegetables (FV)

Eating FV first at the meal ("FVFIRST") may have the added benefit of being a portion-control strategy that can reduce total mealtime calories (Roe et al., 2012; Rolls et al., 2004), as well as making FV taste better because they are eaten when children are most hungry. One advantage of focusing on these three CDC-recommended behaviors is that they can be accomplished in both school and home environments that children experience daily.

BENEFITS OF SCHOOL-BASED PROGRAMS

Health education provided by most schools covers the CDC-recommended behaviors of eating FV, choosing low-fat and low-sugar drinks, and exercising daily. Unfortunately, research suggests that education alone teaches children only **TO KNOW** about these healthy behaviors, but not **TO DO** them, with little impact on their behavior or weight (Contento et al., 1995; Roseman et al., 2010). These healthy behaviors are also targeted by hospital-based clinical programs for overweight children or extreme picky eaters (Paul et al., 2007; Pizzo et al., 2009). However, these programs usually treat one child at a time, which can make children feel different from peers, and behaviors learned in clinic settings may not generalize to children's everyday environments of school and home.

The school-provided lunch gives many children their most consistent source of the FV recommended by the CDC for both overweight children and picky eaters. Unfortunately, as many as 80% of school-children avoid eating the FV provided in their school lunch (Gleason & Suitor, 2000), and without intervention their FV consumption drops by 25% between third and eighth grades (Lytel et al., 2000). Children usually accept fruit more readily than vegetables (Baxter & Thompson, 2002; Edwards & Hartwell, 2002), probably because of the greater sweetness of fruit (Birch, 1979). However, when other more high-fat or high-sugar foods are included in school lunch, children are even less likely to eat the healthy FV (Cullen et al., 2000).

Because most American children have school lunch and recess five days per week for nine months of the year (James et al., 1996), school-based programs offer a unique opportunity for interventions to guide many children to develop healthy behaviors while in their everyday environments and while in the company of their peers. However, most of the existing school-based programs provide poorly documented changes in children's behaviors and weight (Blanchette & Brug, 2005; Budd & Volpe, 2006; Howerton et al., 2007; Knai et al., 2006; Roseman et al., 2010), most of them use time-consuming procedures that may be unacceptable to busy school staff and parents (Bauer et al., 2004; Contento et al., 1995), and none of them estimate program costs.

PAST SCHOOL PROGRAMS TO IMPROVE CHILDREN'S HEALTHY BEHAVIORS

Many past school programs have relied on children's or parents' self-report of behavior or weight changes to evaluate their effectiveness, but a few programs have used more valid direct observation and measurement of changes. For example, increased FV consumption has been documented by the FOOD DUDES (Horne et al., 1995), GIMME-5 (Baranowski et al., 2000), 5-A-DAY-POWER-PLUS (Perry et al., 1998, 2004), KNOW YOUR BODY (Resnicow et al., 1992), and HIGH-5 (Reynolds et al., 2000). Increased exercise has been documented by the PLAY program (Pangrazi et al., 2003). Reduction in BMI% scores have been documented by the SMART program (Robinson, 1999), but the program uses compulsory exercise rather than guiding children to choose more exercise.

Unfortunately, even these programs that are effective for improving children's healthy behavior include complex procedures (Bauer et al., 2004; Contento et al., 1995) that may include purchase of special videos, teachers adding health curricula, cafeteria staff changing lunch menus, physical education instructors supervising exercise sessions, nurses organizing special health presentations, office staff making daily loudspeaker announcements, and parents doing health activities with their children at home. Also, few programs have evaluated acceptability ratings from those involved (children, parents, school staff), which can affect the success of long-term program application.

GOALS OF THE KID'S CHOICE PROGRAM (KCP)

The Kid's Choice Program (KCP) was designed as a new and improved school-based program to encourage children's healthy behaviors and reduce child obesity. The first KCP goal was to increase three CDC-recommended behaviors that could occur in both the children's school and home environments: (1) FV-FIRST = eat FV first during meals, (2) HDRINK = choose low-fat and low-sugar healthy drinks, and (3) EXERCISE = show body movement daily. The second KCP goal was to improve children's preference ratings for these healthy behaviors, especially eating FV, the food group most neglected by picky eaters. The third KCP goal was to reduce BMI% scores for overweight children as an intervention against child obesity and to maintain or reduce BMI% scores for normal-weight children as a prevention against child obesity.

UNIQUE FEATURES OF THE KCP

The KCP was developed to encourage children to choose healthy behaviors that improve their diet quality and weight management, but using methods that improve upon those of past school-based programs. For example, the KCP uses simple school procedures, its effectiveness has been documented with direct observation and measurement of healthy behaviors and weight status for thousands of elementary schoolchildren, and its costs and acceptance ratings by children, parents, and school staff have been evaluated and published (Hendy et al., 2005, 2007, 2011, 2013; Hendy, Williams, Camise, Rahn, et al., 2009). (Please see Textbox 1.3 for suggested readings on KCP effectiveness.)

TEXTBOX 1.3 READINGS ON KCP EFFECTIVENESS

Hendy, H. M., Williams, K. E., & Camise, T. S. (2005). "Kid's Choice" school lunch program increases children's fruit and vegetable acceptance. *Appetite, 45,* 250–263.

Hendy, H. M., Williams, K. E., & Camise, T. S. (2011). Kid's Choice Program improves weight management behaviors and weight status in school children. *Appetite, 56,* 484–494.

Hendy, H. M., Williams, K. E., & Camise, T. S. (in press). Kid's Choice Program increases healthy food choices by fussy-eating children during school lunch. In F. Columbus (Ed.), *Healthy eating: Nutrition, techniques, and benefits.* Hauppauge, NY: Nova Science Publishers.

Hendy, H. M., Williams, K. E., Camise, T. S., Alderman, S., Ivy, J., & Reed, J. (2007). Overweight and average-weight children equally responsive to "Kid's Choice Program" to increase fruit and vegetable consumption. *Appetite, 49,* 683–686.

Hendy, H. M., Williams, K. E., Camise, T. S., Rahn, D., Costigan, C., Gaskins, S., & Moyer, C. (2009). Kid's Choice Program improves two weight management behaviors in school children. In Columbus, F. (Ed.), *Vegetables and health.* Hauppauge, NY: Nova Science Publications.

The KCP was developed by our unique team of professionals, each with over 20 years of experience improving the health and well-being of young children. Our team includes a past elementary school principal, a hospital clinician who specializes in working with parents to improve their children's severe picky eating, and a research psychologist who specializes in testing school programs to improve children's healthy behaviors. We designed the KCP to be an evidence-based, easy-to-use, well-accepted, and low-cost school program to improve children's healthy behaviors in their everyday environments, while in the company of their peers.

The KCP has unique features not included in other school-based programs:

- It targets specific and simple-to-understand healthy behaviors:
  o FVFIRST = eat 1/8 cup FV (size of a ping-pong ball) in first 10 minutes of lunch
  o HDRINK = choose low-fat, low-sugar healthy drink
  o EXERCISE = move the body in first 10 minutes of recess
- It uses three simple school procedures that do not impinge on instructional time
  o NAMETAGS are worn by children during lunch and recess
  o TOKEN REWARDS are given if children choose healthy behaviors
  o REWARD DAYS are presented weekly to trade tokens for small prizes
- It is low in cost at $2 per child per month (or less)
- It can be delivered by small teams of 2–4 volunteers (such as parents)
- It is well accepted by children, parents, and school staff (see Textbox 1.4.)
- It is documented to increase children's healthy behaviors (FV-FIRST, HDRINK, EXERCISE)
- It is documented to increase healthy food choices by picky eaters
- It is documented to increase children's preferences for these healthy behaviors
- It is documented to decrease BMI% scores for overweight children
- It is documented to decrease or maintain BMI% scores for nor-mal-weight children

The unique features of the KCP make it ideal for long-term ap-plication in schools. Small teams of 2–4 parent volunteers can be trained in five minutes to deliver the program at lunch and recess, which eliminates additional work for school staff. The low cost of the KCP is maintained because most supplies are readily available at school (such as FV served for school lunch, index cards and yarn for nametags, hole-punchers to deliver token rewards). Also, the small prizes used for Reward Day are readily available in bulk from a variety of vendors, and their cost can be reduced by community-donated prizes, school fund-drives, and state or federal grants.

TEXTBOX 1.4 QUOTES FROM PARENTS AND SCHOOL STAFF ABOUT KCP

- "My daughter enjoyed being part of this program. It reinforced what I try to do at home. Thank you!"
- "The program conveyed age-appropriate information and held my child's interest throughout."
- "We thought it was a great way to encourage exercise and healthy eating."

PURPOSE AND ORGANIZATION OF THE KCP GUIDE

The purpose of the KCP Guide is to provide all information needed by school leaders (such as principals, school nurses, parent-teacher organizations) to apply the KCP for children at their school. Once implemented, the KCP can continue independently without additional work from the principal or other school staff, requiring only the small teams of parent volunteers to deliver the program during lunch and recess.

The KCP Guide is organized to describe first the background research that served as the foundation of the KCP (Chapter 2), then the research documenting KCP effectiveness for improving children's healthy behaviors and weight (Chapter 3). The next four chapters describe how to apply the program with the three KCP school procedures at lunch and recess (Chapter 4), the KCP personnel involved (Chapter 5), the KCP materials and costs (Chapter 6), and (optionally) methods for documenting effectiveness of the KCP for improving healthy behaviors and weight status for children at your school (Chapter 7). The handbook also includes a chapter on other parent mealtime actions (Chapter 8) useful at home to encourage children to develop healthy eating patterns, as well as guidelines for when to seek professional help (Chapter 9). Finally, the KCP Guide ends with references, author biographies, and acknowledgments.

2

DEVELOPMENT OF CHILDREN'S HEALTH BEHAVIORS

Development of the Kid's Choice Program relied heavily on past theory and research on how children acquire their health-related behaviors, especially their eating habits. In this section, we summarize some of the past work that guided us to determine the most promising components of the KCP.

EARLY DEVELOPMENT OF CHILDREN'S EATING HABITS

Long before children enter school, they have already established many of their eating habits, including patterns of their most preferred and non-preferred foods. Development of these food preferences depends upon many biological and environmental factors. Even prior to birth, children's taste and olfactory systems are functioning, and they can experience the flavors of foods eaten by their mothers through the amniotic fluid. For example, children's exposure to FV flavors before birth has been found to be associated with their willingness to eat FV during infancy (Mennella et al., 2001). While this early prenatal learning can increase children's preference for a wider range of foods, there is (unfortunately!) a developmental milestone that occurs in young children that has been called "food neophobia," or an avoidance of novel foods (Cooke, 2007).

Neophobia usually starts between 18 and 24 months of age, limiting the development of diet variety and giving toddlers the often well-deserved reputation of being picky eaters (Falciglia et al., 2000; Skinner et al., 2002). While neophobia is often described as a "phase," one study found that 40% of children who were picky eaters at age 5 remained picky eaters at age 14 (McDermott et al., 2010), suggesting that children may not always "grow out of it" and that active measures are needed to improve children's diet quality.

Studies from around the world suggest that children often prefer foods of questionable nutritional value, which presents their parents, educators, and health care providers a challenge in guiding them toward healthier eating habits. As young as 2 years of age, American children's favorite foods tend to be high-fat and high-sugar foods (such as pizza, fried chicken, French fries, potato chips, chocolate chip cookies, and soda), and their least favorite foods tend to be vegetables (ADA, 2000; Gleason & Suitor, 2000; Skinner et al., 2002). Unfortunately, these patterns are seen in children from France (Bellisle et al., 2000), Great Britain (Cooke & Wardle, 2005), Germany (Diehl, 1999), and Spain (Perez-Rodrigo et al., 2003). Because we know that food preferences are directly related to food selection (Drewnowski, 1997), these natural food preferences of children do not usually lead them to a healthy diet without some guidance.

THEORIES OF HOW CHILDREN CHANGE HEALTH BEHAVIORS

Components of the KCP were guided by three well-tested theories of behavior change. Social Cognitive Theory (Bandura, 1997) suggests that children's confidence (or self-efficacy) to perform any new behavior, including health-related behaviors, would be enhanced by small *repeated experiences* with the behavior. It also proposes that getting the behavior started would be enhanced by offers of *small rewards* as incentives. Both Social Cognitive Theory (Bandura, 1997) and Group Socialization Theory (Harris, 1995) propose further that the development of a new behavior in children would be encouraged by the presence of many *peer models*. Finally, Self Determination Theory (Deci & Ryan, 1985) suggests that "intrinsic motivation" to perform any new behavior would be enhanced by *perceived choices* surrounding the behavior (please see textbox 2.1).

THE ROLE OF REPEATED EXPERIENCE

A large and growing research literature documents the importance of repeated experience in the development of children's food preferences (Cooke, 2007). For example, infants repeatedly given tastes of a pureed vegetable increased their acceptance of it, and this acceptance lasted over a period of nine months (Maier et al., 2007). Also, repeated exposure to FV during weaning was found to be associated with more FV consumption when the children were preschoolers (Cooke et al., 2004). More specifically, laboratory research has shown that to increase food preference, children need to *taste* the food on approximately 8 to 10 occasions, rather than just look at the food (Birch & Marlin, 1982; Birch et al., 1987; Sullivan & Birch, 1990, 1994; Wardle et al., 2003).

Studies conducted in children's natural environments have also demonstrated that repeated taste exposure can increase diet variety. When parents asked their children to taste a vegetable daily in the home over a 14-day period, these children reported liking this food more than children who received no exposure but just educational information about the food (Wardle et al., 2003). This study also found that the children exposed to the one food repeatedly were also more willing to try other new foods that were not part of the research. Similarly, children in feeding clinics who learn acceptance of one new healthy food often show generalization to other new healthy foods (Williams, Paul, Pizzo, and Riegel 2008).

Unfortunately, even though we know that approximately 8 to 10 repeated exposures to new foods can increase children's diet variety, we also know that parents tend to give up after 3 to 5 exposures (Carruth et al., 1998). Alternatively, school lunches may be an excellent place to increase the diet variety of picky eaters because the foods included on lunch menus tend to be served repeatedly across the course of a school year. It may also be easier to encourage children to taste new foods in school settings where same-aged peers are present and also trying these foods.

THE ROLE OF REWARDS

In their work with children who are extreme picky eaters as well as children with a range of other feeding problems, clinicians have long included positive reinforcement (or the offer of rewards) as one of many components in their interventions. In a review of the intervention literature on food refusal, which is the most severe form of childhood feeding disorder, positive reinforcement was the most widely used intervention component, being included in 37 of 38 studies reviewed (Williams et al., 2010). The type of rewards used in these studies varied, with some studies using verbal praise, tangible rewards, or access to preferred activities. The use of rewards is also extensive in clinical interventions for the eating problems of children with autism spectrum disorders (Williams & Seiverling, 2010).

While the use of positive reinforcement has a long history in the field of education, and especially special education, the use of rewards or incentives is not without controversy (Kohn, 1993). For example, many studies document that offering children small rewards (such as verbal praise, stickers, access to favorite activities) can increase their consumption of FV (Baranowski et al., 2000; Cooke et al., 2011; Davis et al., 2000; Hendy, 1999; Horne et al., 1995, 2011; Perry et al., 1998; Reynolds et al., 2000; Stark et al., 1986; Story et al., 2000). However, other studies suggest that if the reward is a favorite *food*, children may later show increased preference for the food given as a reward and decreased preference for the food they had to eat to get it (Birch et al., 1982, 1984; Newman & Taylor, 1992).

These patterns have been called the "over-justification effect" (Lepper et al., 1973) and they have been explained in two ways.

One idea for why preference for a rewarded food may drop is a cognitive explanation suggesting that children think that if they must be offered a favorite food in order to eat another food ("over-justification" for eating it), it must be because the rewarded food tastes bad and they will not like it (Newman & Layton, 1984; Newman & Taylor, 1992). Another view is a satiation explanation suggesting that if the offer of any type of reward for eating a food pushes consumption of that food past the point of satiation, children will begin to dislike the food (Hendy et al., 2005). This happens to us all of the time. Even if pizza is your favorite food, if you eat pizza several meals or days in a row, you become satiated on pizza.

Fortunately, such drops in preference for rewarded foods may be avoided if children are only asked to eat small amounts of food, and if only small and delayed rewards are offered (Eisenberger & Cameron, 1996; Hendy et al., 2005, 2007; Horne et al., 1995). The use of such small and delayed reward is done by offering children small "tokens" immediately after eating healthy foods, then later allowing them to trade tokens for small non-food prizes. Such token reward programs may improve both consumption and preference for healthy foods because they avoid food satiation, make rewards less prominent, and give children time to discover pleasant properties of the foods themselves (Hitt et al., 1992; Newman & Layton, 1984).

THE ROLE OF PEER MODELING

The use of modeling to teach children new behaviors has been a staple in the field of education, with over 70 years of research showing its effectiveness for influencing children's eating behavior. Two early studies showed that peer modeling could increase children's food consumption, with effects lasting until one year later, even when the peer model was not present (Duncker, 1938; Marinho, 1942). Adult modeling can also increase children's food consumption (Harper & Sanders, 1975; Hendy, 2002), especially if adults use "enthusiastic modeling" by saying how good food tastes (Hendy & Raudenbush, 2000). However, when directly competing with peer models, the effectiveness of adult models fades (Hendy & Raudenbush, 2000).

THE ROLE OF PERCEIVED CHOICES

During focus group interviews to determine factors associated with children's willingness to try new lunch foods, children themselves report that they want "choices" (James et al., 1996; Marples & Spillman, 1995). Experimental research has also documented that offering children some very simple "choices" during school lunch can increase their FV consumption (Hendy, 1999; Perry et al., 2004), but its effects on food consumption and preference ratings can depend on the details of how such "choices" are presented.

For example, one experimental study found that when teachers verbally offered children the choice of whether or not to eat a new food during lunch (e.g., "Do you want any of this mango?"), children increased food consumption above mere exposure to the food without comment (Hendy, 1999). However, questionnaire data for both average-developing children and feeding-clinic children suggest that when parents become too permissive with food choices (such as by preparing "special meals" for their children that are different from the shared family meal), children tend to continue with their picky eating patterns and fail to develop a healthy variety in their diets (Hendy et al., 2010; Hendy, Williams, Camise, Eckman, Hedemann, 2009; Timimi et al., 1997).

At the other extreme, giving children no food choice by forbidding their favorite high-fat, high-sugar, and high-salt snack foods may backfire and result in overconsumption of these foods later when children have the opportunity (Baughcum et al., 2001; Birch et al., 2001; Fisher & Birch, 1999). Or, giving children no food choice by forcing them to eat disliked foods with the threat of punishment may result in "learned taste aversions" that can last a lifetime (Batsell et al., 2002; Galloway et al., 2005; Rolls et al., 1981; Rozin, 1986; Sanders et al., 1993).

SELECTION OF THE KCP TARGET BEHAVIOR OF EATING FV FIRST DURING MEALS

One target behavior of the Kid's Choice Program was not only to increase children's FV consumption, as recommended by the CDC, but to increase their consumption of FV *first* during meals ("FV-FIRST"). (See Photo 2.1.) This goal was selected because of several studies showing that a "first course" of low-calorie food can serve as a portion-control strategy that decreases total calories consumed at that meal. For example, two studies found that when adults ate salad *before* the rest of their meal, they consumed up to 12% fewer calories during that meal (Roe et al., 2012; Rolls et al., 2004). This same research showed that when salads were eaten *with* the meal, this decrease in caloric density did not occur. Similar results have been found when individuals ate fruit (Flood-Obbagy & Rolls, 2009) before other foods during the meal.

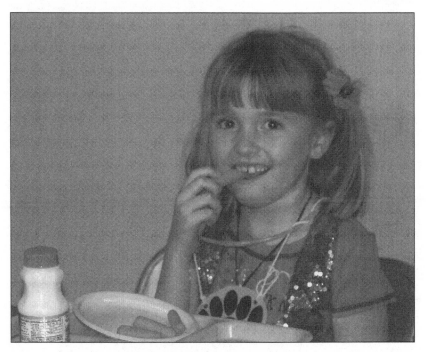

Photo 2.1 Eat Fruit or Vegetables First at Lunch (FVFIRST)

SELECTION OF THE KCP TARGET BEHAVIOR OF CHOOSING HEALTHY DRINKS

Another KCP target behavior was the CDC-recommended increase in children's consumption of low-fat, low-sugar healthy drinks such as skim milk, low-fat milk, 100% juice, or water ("HDRINK"). (See Photo 2.2.) Research suggests that calories consumed in liquids tend to be "stealthy" and produce no adjustments in later mealtime calories consumed (DiMeglio & Mattes, 2000). This effect means that an unnoticed reduction in total calories can be produced when low-fat, low-sugar drinks are chosen, with a gradual reduction in children's BMI% scores. For example, if children switch from their usual school lunch drink of a half pint of 2%-fat sweetened chocolate milk (195 kcal) to a half pint of skim milk (86 kcal), those children would consume 545 fewer calories per week.

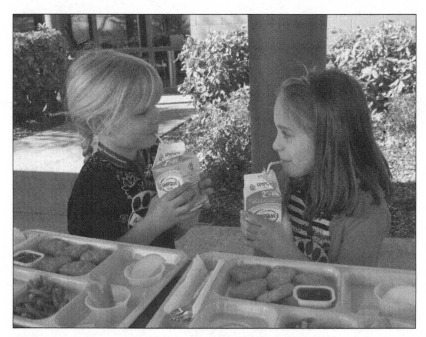

Photo 2.2 Choose Low-Fat, Low-Sugar Healthy Drinks (HDRINK)

SELECTION OF THE KCP TARGET BEHAVIOR OF EXERCISE

The third KCP target behavior was the CDC-recommended increase of children's exercise behavior ("EXERCISE"). (See Photo 2.3.) This goal was selected because, as might be expected, children who are obese have been found to engage in less physical activity and more sedentary behaviors (e.g., television viewing) than non-obese children (Trost et al., 2001), with the children who engage in the least physical activity and the most sedentary behavior being the most overweight (Andersen et al., 1998). One study found that each hour of moderate to vigorous exercise per day decreased the risk of obesity by 10%. (Hernandez et al., 1999).

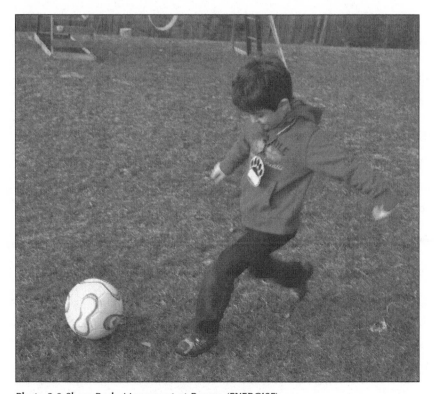

Photo 2.3 Show Body Movement at Recess (EXERCISE)

TEXTBOX 2.1 READINGS ON THEORY OF CHILDREN'S BEHAVIOR CHANGE

Bandura, A. (1997). *Self-efficacy: The exercise of control.* New York: Freeman & Company.

Cooke, L. J., Chambers, L. C., Afiez, E. V., Croker, H. A., Boniface, D., Yeomans, M. R., & Wardle, J. (2011). Eating for pleasure or profit: The effect of incentives on children's enjoyment of vegetables. *Psychological Science, 22,* 190–196.

Deci, E. L., & Ryan, R. M. (1985). *Intrinsic motivation and self determination in human behavior.* New York: Plenum.

Eisenberger, R., & Cameron, J. (1996). Detrimental effects of reward. *American Psychologist, 51,* 1153–1166.

Harris, J. R. (1995). Where is the child's environment? A group socialization theory of development. *Psychological Review, 102,* 458–489.

Adult guided exercise has often been included in child obesity interventions. For example, one study randomly assigned 82 obese children to one of two six-week interventions that guided them either in dietary changes alone or dietary changes plus exercise (Woo et al., 2004). While both groups improved their weight status, the diet-plus-exercise group showed the most improvement in body fat composition and blood lipids. However, the exercise shown by the children in this study was *required* and guided by adults, rather than being *chosen* by the children, as is the goal for the Kid's Choice Program. We believe that when children are encouraged to *choose* exercise, it is more likely to generalize to other contexts.

Some school-based programs for child weight management have also included exercise, but the children are typically *required* to show body movement, rather than *choosing* to do so. For example, children in one school-based study were randomly assigned to an exercise group or a control group (Mo-suwan et al., 1998). In the exercise group, children were guided by adults to walk for 15 minutes in the morning and to do aerobic dance for 20 minutes in the afternoon three days per week for 29 weeks. Results showed that the prevalence of obesity decreased more in the exercise group when compared to the control group. However, because children did not *choose* the exercise, they may have been less likely to enjoy it or continue it.

3

RESEARCH DOCUMENTING KCP EFFECTIVENESS

In this chapter, we describe research we conducted that documented effectiveness of the KCP applications with 1000-plus children including first through fourth graders, boys and girls, picky eaters, overweight and normal-weight children (Hendy et al., 2005, 2007, 2011, 2012; Hendy, Williams, Camise, Rahn, et al., 2009). Our research demonstrates that in one- to three-month applications, the KCP improves children's healthy behaviors (such as FVFIRST, HDRINK, EXERCISE), children's preference ratings for these healthy behaviors, and children's weight status as measured by their BMI% scores. Our research also examines which KCP components were effective for changing the children's healthy behavior (token reward, peer modeling), and whether small teams of 2–4 parent volunteers could validly and effectively deliver the KCP. Finally, our research documents KCP acceptability ratings from children, parents, and school staff, as well as KCP costs (in U.S. dollars) per child per month of program application.

KCP-PRODUCED CHANGES IN CHILDREN'S HEALTHY BEHAVIORS

One KCP goal was to improve children's CDC-recommended healthy behaviors for weight management, and this goal was approached in four KCP applications with different sets of elementary schoolchildren. The first KCP application was made with 346 first- through fourth-grade children (Hendy et al., 2005, 2007). After one month of baseline lunch observations of children's consumption of fruit and vegetables, children were randomly assigned for one month to either a KCP-FRUIT group or a KCP-VEGETABLE group that earned stars punched in nametags for eating either 1/8 cup fruit or vegetables (the size of a ping-pong ball). Weekly Reward Days let children trade stars for small prizes. Results showed that children increased consumption of the food type rewarded, both in overweight and normal-weight children.

The second KCP application was made at another school with 320 first- through third-grade children (Hendy et al., in press; Hendy, Williams, Camise, Rahn, et al., 2009). After one month of baseline lunch observations, children were randomly assigned for one month to one of two groups: (1) KCP Group earned stars punched into nametags for "Good Health Behaviors" (FVFIRST, HDRINK, FOUR FOODS = eating 1/8 cup of FV, grains, meat/meat substitutes, milk). (2) Control group earned stars for "Good Citizenship Behaviors" (talking quietly, keeping lunch area clean, respecting others by not touching them or their things). Weekly Reward Days let children trade stars for small prizes. Results showed that KCP Group children (even "picky eaters" who had never eaten FV in baseline) increased their FVFIRST, HDRINKS, and FOUR FOODS during school lunch.

The third KCP application was made at another school with 382 first- through fourth-grade children (Hendy et al., 2011). After one month of baseline lunch observations, pedometer records, and BMI% scores measured by the school nurse, children were randomly assigned for three months to one of two groups: (1) KCP Group earned stars for "Good Health Behaviors" (FVFIRST, HDRINK, EX-

ERCISE = body movement recorded as pedometer steps). (2) Control group earned stars for "Good Citizenship Behaviors" (defined as in the second KCP application). Weekly Reward Days allowed children to trade stars for small prizes. Results showed that KCP Group children (even those with home-packed lunches) increased their healthy behaviors (FVFIRST, HDRINKS, EXERCISE). (See Figure 3.1.)

We also used this third KCP application to examine whether the two program components (token rewards, peer models) had separate effects on the children's healthy behaviors (FVFIRST, HDRINK, EXERCISE). Results demonstrated that after one month of KCP application, peer modeling had established separate and significant effects on children's healthy behaviors, above and beyond effects of the token rewards. These results suggest that school leaders may "thin" the number of Reward Days after one month, both to reduce costs and to move children toward "intrinsic" motivation for demonstrating the healthy behaviors.

The fourth KCP application was made with 111 second- and third-grade children who had participated in the third KCP application the year before (Hendy et al., 2011). After one week of baseline lunch observations for three healthy behaviors (eating 1/8 cup FV during the first 10 minutes of lunch, choosing HDRINK, and EXERCISE = body movement recorded as the number of 5,000 pedometer steps since the previous observed lunch), all children were assigned to KCP conditions for one week, during which they earned a star for each healthy behavior, delivered by the 2–4 parent volunteers each day (Monday, Wednesday, Friday). The Reward Day on Friday was presented by 2 parent volunteers.

Training of the parent volunteers required less than five minutes. (See Chapter 5 for details of the training of parent volunteers.) To check validity of the parent volunteers' lunch observations, trained research assistants walked ahead of each volunteer to record FVFIRST, HDRINK, and EXERCISE, then the volunteer verbalized her decision for each child's star delivery, and the observer noted their agreement. For 25 children simultaneously observed in this manner, mean agreement scores were 100% for FVFIRST, 95% for HDRINK,

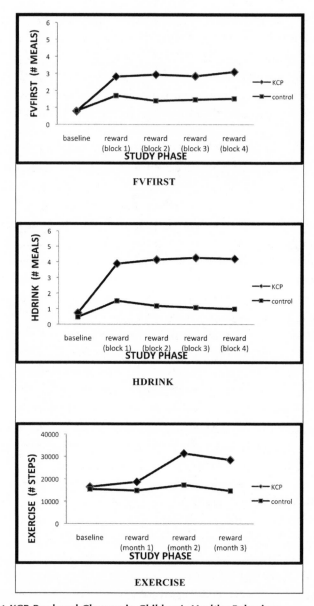

Figure 3.1 KCP-Produced Changes in Children's Healthy Behaviors
Changes in three weight management behaviors from one month of baseline conditions through
three months of KCP conditions for 346 children randomly assigned to either a KCP group or a
control group. FVFIRST = eating FV first during school lunch, HDRINK = choosing low-fat and
low-sugar healthy drinks, EXERCISE = body movement recorded as steps on a pedometer (Hendy
et al., 2011). (Permission for figures from Elsevier Publishing.)

and 90% for EXERCISE. Results from this brief KCP application by parent volunteers showed children increased all three behaviors from baseline to KCP conditions.

KCP-PRODUCED CHANGES IN CHILDREN'S PREFERENCE FOR HEALTHY BEHAVIORS

Another KCP goal was to increase children's preference ratings for healthy behaviors, with special focus on FV preferences because they represent the food groups most rejected by picky eaters (Carruth et al., 2004; Dovey et al., 2008; Galloway et al., 2005). To examine changes in children's FRUIT and VEGETABLE preference ratings from baseline conditions to follow-up conditions after the first KCP application described above, we conducted interviews with 158 children whose parents gave permission to do so (Hendy et al., 2005).

Children pointed to a laminated card with three cartoon faces (1 = frowning face, "I don't like it," 2 = neutral face, "It is just OK," 3 = smiling face, "I like it") to report how much they liked eight common fruits and eight common vegetables, with the mean rating used as the preference score. Results showed that children's fruit and vegetable preference scores increased from baseline to after the one-month KCP application. Similar increases in FV preferences were found for picky eaters who had completely rejected FV in baseline conditions before the second KCP application described above (Hendy et al., 2012).

KCP-PRODUCED CHANGES IN WEIGHT FOR OVER-WEIGHT AND NORMAL-WEIGHT CHILDREN

One of the most important KCP goals was to decrease BMI% scores for overweight children (as a child obesity intervention) and to decrease or maintain BMI% scores for normal-weight children (as a child obesity prevention). During the third KCP application described above, the school nurse provided children's BMI% scores using CDC standards. We found that only after the three-month KCP application did 112 overweight children (with initial BMI% above 85%) and 200 normal-weight children (with initial BMI% between 10% and 85%) show drops in their BMI% scores, while still avoiding underweight BMI% scores under 10%. The mean BMI% drop was 2.6% for overweight children and 2.4% for normal-weight children. These results suggest the KCP is effective for both *intervention* and *prevention* of child overweight. (See Figure 3.2.)

KCP ACCEPTABILITY RATINGS BY CHILDREN, PARENTS, AND SCHOOL STAFF

After the second KCP application described above, we gathered program acceptability ratings from 154 children using brief interviews, and from 151 parents using brief questionnaires (Hendy, Williams, Camise, Rahn, et al., 2009). Children again used the three cartoon faces (1 = frowning face, 2 = neutral face, 3 = smiling face) to report how much they liked the KCP, and parents used a five-point rating (from 1 = not at all to 5 = very much) for how acceptable the KCP would be "as an ongoing program done throughout the school year." Results showed that children gave a mean KCP acceptability score of 2.9 using their three-point rating, and that parents gave a mean KCP acceptability score of 4.4 using their five-point rating.

After the third KCP application described above, we gathered program acceptability ratings from 31 school staff using brief questionnaires (Hendy et al., 2011). School staff included the principal, secretaries, school nurse, custodians, cafeteria staff, physical education instructors, first- through fourth-grade teachers, and teachers' aides. They were asked to use a five-point rating (from 1 = not at all to 5 = very much) for how acceptable the KCP would be "for long-term application throughout the school year."

Results showed that that school staff gave a mean KCP acceptability score of 3.8 using their five-point rating. Specific program options *most liked* by school staff were targeting the three weight management behaviors (FVFIRST, HDRINK, EXERCISE), having children wear nametags, using star-shaped holes in nametags as

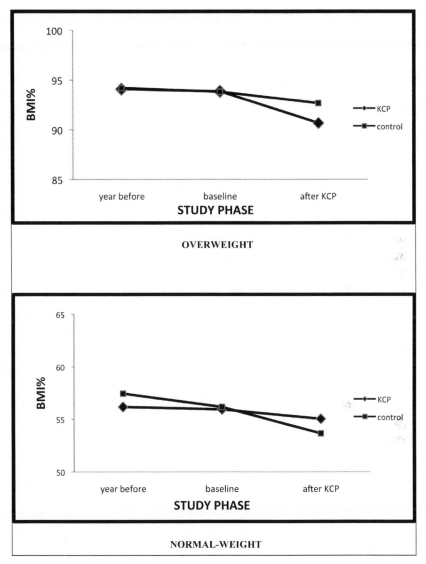

Figure 3.2 KCP-Produced Changes in Children's Weight Status
Changes in children's BMI% scores from the school year before KCP application, to base-line conditions immediately before KCP application, to two weeks after KCP application for 112 overweight children (with BMI% over 85th percentile) and 200 average-weight children (with BMI% scores between 10th and 85th percentile). Both overweight and normal-weight children who received the KCP showed significant drops in BMI% (while avoiding underweight BMI% values under 10th percentile), suggesting that the KCP is effective for both *intervention* and *prevention* of child obesity (Hendy et al., 2011). (Permission for figures from Elsevier Publishing.)

token rewards, presenting weekly Reward Days, including Parent Records to report children's behaviors at home, and having parent volunteers deliver the program. Program options *least liked* by school staff were using pedometers to record exercise and having busy school staff deliver the program themselves rather than parent volunteers.

KCP COSTS PER CHILD PER MONTH OF APPLICATION

In the second and third KCP applications described above (Hendy et al., 2011; Hendy, Williams, Camise, Rahn, et al., 2009), we documented that the KCP costs approximately US$2 per child per month of application, with these funds used to cover the small prizes used for Reward Days. These costs can be reduced by community-donated prizes, school fund-drives, and state or federal wellness grants. (See Chapter 6 for more information on KCP materials and costs.) All other supplies used for KCP applications are already available at most schools, such as the FV and healthy drink options used at lunch, the exercise options used at recess, and the index cards, yarn, and hole-punchers used for nametags and token rewards.

KCP APPLICATION:
SCHOOL PROCEDURES

THREE SIMPLE KCP SCHOOL PROCEDURES

We designed the Kid's Choice Program (KCP) to include only three simple school procedures that teach children how **TO DO** healthy behaviors, rather than just **TO KNOW** about them. Our goal was that these simple procedures could be applied throughout the school year because they are easy-to-use, they do not impinge upon instructional time, they are low in cost (at less than US$2 per child per month), they use mostly available school supplies, they can be delivered by small teams of 2–4 volunteers, and they are well accepted by children, parents, and school staff. The three simple school procedures of the KCP include:

- Nametags worn by children during lunch and recess
- Token rewards given when children choose healthy behaviors:
  - o FVFIRST = eat 1/8 cup FV (size of a ping-pong ball) in first 10 minutes of lunch
  - o HDRINK = choose low-fat, low-sugar healthy drink for lunch
  - o EXERCISE = move the body in first 10 minutes of recess
- Reward days presented weekly to trade tokens for small prizes

DELIVERY OF TOKEN REWARDS DURING LUNCH AND RECESS

We deliver the KCP three days a week (e.g., Monday, Wednesday, Friday) because that provides a good balance between giving children frequent and repeated experience with the new, healthy behaviors but without over-presenting the program so that they become tired of it. Children wear nametags (only at lunch and recess) so that token rewards earned for their healthy behavior choices can be delivered to them individually (such as holes punched into the nametags). We use nametag necklaces so that children's hands can remain free during lunch and recess. (See Chapter 6 for instructions on making nametags.)

We use star-shaped holes punched into nametags as the token reward for children's healthy choices, but many other options are possible. (See Photo 4.1.) Tokens work best when they can be immediately applied to the nametags so that children's hands remain free and when they would not be easily broken or lost. (See Chapter 6 for a list of possible token rewards to use instead of the star-shaped holes.)

During school lunch (Monday, Wednesday, Friday), the KCP volunteers wait until children have been seated with their school-provided lunches for 10 minutes, then they deliver token rewards as star-shaped hole punches in the children's nametags for each healthy behavior they have chosen. For example, if a child eats 1/8 cup of FVFIRST sometime during the first 10 minutes of lunch (such as by eating a ping-pong ball size of salad, green beans, or orange), he/she would get one star. If the child chose a HDRINK that was low-fat and low-sugar (such as 1% or 2% white milk, skim milk, 100% orange juice, or water), he/she would get one star.

For children with home-packed lunches, the same procedures and the same definitions of FVFIRST and HDRINK are used. So that their healthy food choices can be seen more easily, children with home-packed lunches are asked by KCP volunteers at the beginning of lunch to remove all items from their lunch bags or boxes.

During school recess (Monday, Wednesday, Friday), the KCP volunteers wait until 10 minutes of recess have elapsed. Then, they give children one token (such as a hole punch in their

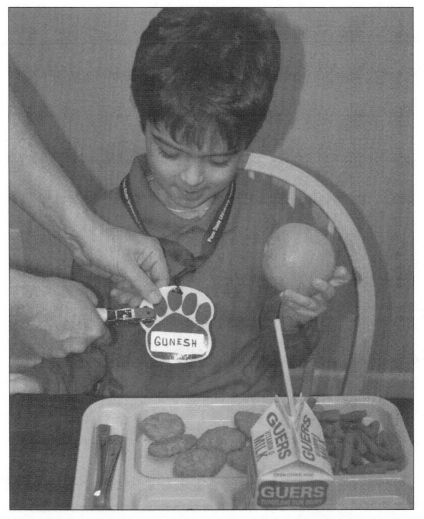

Photo 4.1 Token Reward when Children Choose Healthy Behaviors

nametags, a sticker, or some other token reward) if they show EXERCISE (body movement) throughout the first 10 minutes of recess. For example, if a child walked with a friend, ran in a game of tag, kicked a soccer ball around, and/or played basketball for the first 10 minutes of recess, the child would receive one star-shaped hole in his/her nametag.

Each school can choose the specific FVFIRST and HDRINK options for children during school lunch. Also, many options can be found to provide children with EXERCISE during school recess. (See Textbox 4.1.)

DELIVERY OF WEEKLY REWARD DAY

Reward Day is presented at the end of the week (Friday), when children may trade a specified number of tokens for one small prize. The advantage of using a slightly delayed Reward Day is that it takes the children's focus off prizes and allows them to discover positive

---

TEXTBOX 4.1 WHICH HEALTHY BEHAVIOR OPTIONS FOR YOUR SCHOOL?

FVFIRST choices available during school lunch:

___ banana	___ baby carrots	___ cooked green beans
___ apple	___ cherry tomatoes	___ canned peaches
___ orange	___ salad	___ canned pears
___ grapes	___ pineapple	___ cooked peas
___ other _____		

HDRINK choices available during school lunch:

___ skim white milk	___ 100% orange juice
___ 1% fat white milk	___ 100% vegetable juice
___ 2% fat white milk	___ water
___ other _____	

EXERCISE choices available during school recess:

___ walking	___ playing tag
___ playing basketball	___climbing
___ running an obstacle course	___kicking soccer ball
___ jumping rope	___running races
___ other _____	

---

characteristics of the healthy behaviors themselves. ("I didn't know that baby carrots were so sweet and crunchy!" "I was surprised how fun soccer could be!")

We specify the number of tokens needed to earn one prize on Reward Day as a number that is over 75% of the total possible tokens earned during the week. For example, if children can earn three stars each day (one for FVFRIST, one for HDRINK, one for EXERCISE), nine stars are possible per week across the three KCP days, so children with seven stars can trade them for one prize.

On Reward Day, we set up a long table in the cafeteria with four to five plastic bins, each containing one type of small prize. During the last 15 minutes of the 30-minute lunch period, children are called up to the Reward table by classroom, then one KCP volunteer counts the tokens on each child's nametag and uses a different hole-puncher (or sticker) to show the number of small prizes earned and to "cancel out" the used tokens. (Children do not lose any extra tokens they have, which can be saved for the next Reward Day.) A second KCP volunteer standing next to the bins then allows the child 10 seconds to select his/her small prize(s).

To speed up the process, samples of all prizes are placed on the table edge for children to examine, and children are asked not to dig around in the bins, but to point to the selected bin so that the volunteer may take out their chosen prize. After receiving their earned prizes, children return to their seats in the cafeteria. We recommend that favorite foods never be used as prizes on Reward Day because research shows that children will learn to like the reward foods *more* while learning to like the healthy foods eaten to earn them *less*, (Newman and Taylor, 1992). (See Chapter 6 for a list of possible small prizes for Reward Day.)

INTRODUCING KCP TO SCHOOL STAFF, PARENTS, AND CHILDREN

We introduce the KCP to school staff and parents with a two-page description of program goals, procedures, and roles for everyone involved. (See Textbox 4.2.) To introduce children to the KCP, the first step is to distribute the nametag materials to the children's classrooms. Children are simply told by their teachers that the nametags are for a new program their school will have for them, and that they will begin wearing them at lunch and recess on Monday, Wednesday, and Friday.

The second step is to make an announcement during school lunch that their school will begin the KCP to help them learn healthy behaviors during lunch and recess. (See Textbox 4.3.) They can earn stars (or other tokens) for their nametags by choosing each healthy behavior, then once a week (on Friday) they will have a Reward Day to trade seven stars for one small prize. (*Note*: During this introduction to the KCP, we show children sample prizes. After that, we keep prizes out of sight until Reward Day.)

We explain to children that during each KCP lunch, they can earn one star for the first healthy behavior of eating fruits or vegetables during the first 10 minute of lunch (FVFIRST = "eating FV first"), and we show them a ping-pong ball as a sample of how much FV they must eat. During each KCP lunch, children can also earn one star for the second healthy behavior of choosing a healthy drink (HDRINK) that is low-fat and low-sugar, and we show them sample healthy drinks.

We also explain to children that during each KCP recess, they can earn one star for the healthy behavior of EXERCISE during the first 10 minutes of recess. We describe exercise as "body movement" such as walking with a friend, running in a game of tag, climbing on the playground equipment, playing basketball, or kicking a soccer ball around.

MOST EFFECTIVE KCP COMPONENTS

The KCP procedures were designed to be easy to use, low in cost, and well accepted by children and school staff. They were also selected to include four important features that provide the power behind the program and that make it effective for improving children's healthy behaviors, lasting preferences for them, and a healthy weight status. These most effective KCP components include:

- 2+ Choices available for each healthy behavior at lunch and recess
- Small and delayed rewards (tokens) as incentives to try new behaviors
- Small repeated experiences with each healthy behavior
- Many peer models available for the healthy behaviors

VARIATIONS ON KCP APPLICATION AT SCHOOL

Although we developed the KCP by testing its effectiveness for first- through fourth-grade children, the simplicity of the KCP procedures would also be effective for younger children in preschool or kindergarten. For example, our past research found that preschool children will increase their consumption of healthy foods at school lunch if offered small rewards as an incentive to try new foods and if they are surrounded by peers who model healthy food choices (Hendy, 1999, 2002).

Additionally, we believe the KCP would be effective for improving healthy behaviors and weight status in older children if age-appropriate adjustments are made to token rewards and Reward Day prizes. For example, rather than "stars" punched into nametags, older children could receive token rewards as stamps in a "Passport to Good Health" booklet. Rather than crayons, puzzles, and silly hats used as Reward Day prizes, older children might be more interested in music, cosmetics, and passes to school events.

The KCP could also be used to target other healthy behaviors besides the three described in the present handbook (FVFIRST, HDRINK, EXERCISE). For example, we have documented that the KCP increases the meals that fussy eaters eat from the four food groups of fruit or vegetable, grains, milk, and meat or meat substitute (Hendy et al., 2013). Other healthy behaviors the KCP could improve would be eating whole-grain foods instead of refined grains, vitamin-packed sweet potato fries instead of white potato fries, fresh fruit for dessert instead of high-calorie foods, and walking or cycling to or from school instead of traveling in a vehicle (as safety concerns allow).

Schools could vary other KCP features according to the personnel and supplies they have available. Besides the parent volunteers and college students who delivered our four KCP applications, the program could be delivered by school aides, grandparents, or high school students after being trained for five minutes with our KCP volunteer handout. (See Chapter 5 for more information about KCP personnel.)

Although we typically use Monday, Wednesday, and Friday to deliver the KCP at school lunch and recess, other days could be used. However, any reduction in the number of KCP days may reduce the program's effectiveness for improving children's healthy behaviors, preferences for these behaviors, and their healthy weight status.

Additionally, schools could use pedometers to record children's EXERCISE (such as with one token given for each 10,000 steps) rather than using observations of children's body movement during the first 10 minutes of recess. However, we have found that pedometers add significant costs to the KCP application (with an increase from $2 to $7 per child per month) because of the frequency with which they are lost or broken by young children, and they are not well accepted by school staff (Hendy et al., 2011).

TEXTBOX 4.2 SAMPLE LETTER EXPLAINING KCP TO SCHOOL STAFF AND PARENTS

Dear School Staff and Parents:

We will soon begin the Kid's Choice Program (KCP), a school-based program to promote healthy behaviors and reduce child obesity. The KCP targets three weight management behaviors:

(1) FVFIRST-eat 1/8 cup of fruit or vegetables (the size of a ping-pong ball) in the first 10 minutes of meals,

(2) HDRINK-choose low-fat and low-sugar healthy drinks, and

(3) EXERCISE-move the body in the first 10 minutes of recess.

The KCP includes components documented by research to encourage children to develop healthy behaviors. They include offers of small and delayed rewards (token rewards) as incentives for children to try the new healthy behaviors, availability of 2+ choices for each healthy behavior, small daily expectations to gradually develop children's acceptance of the new behaviors, and conditions that encourage the power of peer modeling.

The KCP has unique features in comparison to other programs to reduce child obesity:

- It uses simple school procedures (without consuming instructional time)
- It is low in cost at $2 per child per month (or less)
- It is well accepted by children, parents, and school staff
- It can be delivered by small teams of 2–4 volunteers (such as parents)
- It is documented to increase children's healthy behaviors
- It is documented to increase children's preferences for these healthy behaviors
- It is documented to decrease weight in overweight children (for intervention)
- It is documented to maintain/decrease weight in normal-weight children (for prevention)
- It is documented to increase healthy food choices by picky eaters

For KCP application, each person involved has a very simple role:

Teachers
- Remind children to wear nametags for lunch and recess (Monday, Wednesday, Friday)
- Distribute Parent Records to children (who bring them back on weekly Reward Days)

Cafeteria staff
- Provide 2+ choices of fruit or vegetable for each school lunch
- Provide 2+ choices of low-fat, low-sugar drinks for each school lunch

Custodian
- Set up two tables in cafeteria once each week for Reward Day (Friday)
- Store bins of small prizes for Reward Day in a secure location

School nurse (Optional)
- Measure children's height and weight (for BMI% calculation) before KCP
- Measure children's height and weight (for BMI% calculation) after KCP

Parents (Optional)
- Complete Parent Records of children's healthy choices at home
- Return completed Parent Records with children on weekly Reward Days (Friday)

Children
- Wear nametags for lunch and recess (Monday, Wednesday, Friday)
- Earn token rewards by choosing healthy behaviors (FV-FIRST, HDRINK, EXERCISE)
- Trade token rewards for small prizes each week on Reward Day (Friday)

KCP volunteers
- Give children token rewards for FVFIRST and HDRINK in first 10 minutes of lunch
- Give children token rewards for EXERCISE in first 10 minutes of recess
- Trade children's token rewards for small prizes on weekly Reward Days (Friday)

Please let us know if you have any questions about the Kid's Choice Program for our children!

TEXTBOX 4.3 SAMPLE SCRIPT TO DESCRIBE KCP TO CHILDREN

Hello 1st, 2nd, 3rd, 4th Graders!

We are very excited to begin the Kid's Choice Program (which we call KCP) at our school! The KCP is a reward program that shows children how to have fun with three healthy choices at lunch and recess.

The KCP has three easy steps:

(1) You wear a nametag at school lunch and recess (Monday, Wednesday, Friday)

(2) You earn stars punched in your nametag if you make healthy choices

(3) You can trade 7 stars for one small prize on Reward Day (Friday)

What are the three healthy choices that can earn you stars? Here they are:

EAT FRUIT OR VEGETABLE FIRST (FVFIRST)

This means that you eat 1/8 cup of F or V in the first 10 minutes of lunch.

How much F or V is that? It is the size of a ping-pong ball (shown).

CHOOSE HEALTHY DRINKS (HDRINK)

This means that you choose a low-fat and low-sugar healthy drink for your lunch.

Some examples are skim, 1%, or 2% white milk, water, 100% FV juice (shown).

EXERCISE

This means that you move your body for the first 10 minutes of recess.

Some examples are walking, running, playing tag, basketball, soccer.

You can earn bonus stars if your parents fill out the Parent Records (shown).

Does anybody want to see some of the prizes you can get on Reward Day (shown)?

We hope that you enjoy the Kid's Choice Program to help you have fun with healthy choices!

5

KCP APPLICATION: PERSONNEL

SMALL TEAMS OF VOLUNTEERS CAN DELIVER THE KCP

B ecause school staff are already busy with their many regular duties, we designed the Kid's Choice Program (KCP) to be delivered by small teams of 2–4 volunteers. During lunch three days each week (Monday, Wednesday, Friday), one volunteer can deliver tokens to about 50 children eating the school-provided lunch. For the more varied home-packed lunches, one volunteer can deliver tokens to about 25 children. During recess three days each week (Monday, Wednesday, Friday), one volunteer can deliver tokens to 25–50 children, depending on the size of the recess area and how widely dispersed children become with their chosen activities.

During Reward Day (Friday), 2 volunteers are needed, 1 volunteer to check the number of tokens and prizes earned by each child and another volunteer to hand children their chosen prizes from the five plastic bins. Our experience has shown that the same volunteers can complete the KCP tasks at lunch, recess, and Reward Day, depending on the school's scheduling of these activities.

TRAINING OF KCP VOLUNTEERS

In our own KCP applications, volunteers have been parents recruited through the Parent Teacher Organization (Hendy et al., 2011). Other volunteers could be grandparents, high school students, or college students. Volunteers are given a two-page handout that describes the KCP, a nametag necklace to wear while at school, a star-shaped hole-puncher, and a ping-pong ball (as a visual reminder of 1/8 cup of FV). They are also asked to follow all school safety procedures such as signing-in and signing-out in the school office logbook.

Training the volunteers to complete their tasks at lunch, recess, and Reward Day takes five minutes or less. Their handout reviews the KCP goals, the targeted healthy behaviors, and the three simple school procedures. The handout also lists the specific tasks asked of KCP volunteers at school lunch, recess, and during Reward Day. (See Textbox 5.1.)

ENCOURAGING PARENT PARTICIPATION

Past research suggests that school-based programs are most effective for improving children's healthy behaviors when they include parents and the home environment (Roseman et al., 2010). One way to include parents in the KCP application so that it becomes a true "school-home partnership" for healthier children (Hendy et al., 2011) is for the parents to use the Parent Records to report the three KCP-targeted healthy behaviors that children show at home. (See Textbox 5.2.)

Our Parent Records are small prepared cards on which parents can record their children's healthy behaviors (FVFIRST, HDRINK, EXERCISE) at home for five days per week. Each day has a space in which parents can record whether or not (X = yes, O = no) their children displayed each of the healthy behaviors: FVFIRST—child ate 1/8 cup FV in first 10 minutes of the meal, HDRINK—child chose a low-fat and low-sugar healthy drink, EXERCISE—child showed body movements for 10+ minutes during the day. Children bring these

---

TEXTBOX 5.1 HANDOUT TO TRAIN KCP VOLUNTEERS

DEAR KCP VOLUNTEER:

Thank you for your assistance with the Kid's Choice Program (KCP) at our school! We have prepared for you a KCP nametag necklace to wear during school lunch and recess, a star-shaped hole puncher, and a ping-pong ball as a visual reminder to the children of the amount of FV they are asked to eat to earn a star punched in their nametags.

We provide below some background information about the Kid's Choice Program by reviewing its goals, targeted healthy behaviors, and simple school procedures. Also listed below are the specific tasks for each KCP volunteer at school lunch, recess, and Reward Day.

REVIEW OF KCP GOALS
- increase three healthy *behaviors* in children
- increase children's *preferences* for these healthy behaviors
- decrease *weight* for overweight children, maintain it for normal-weight children

A REVIEW OF KCP-TARGETED HEALTHY BEHAVIORS
- FVFIRST = child eats 1/8 cup FV in first 10 minutes of lunch (but not potatoes)
- HDRINK = child chooses low-fat and low-sugar healthy drink (skim or low-fat white milk, water, 100% juice)
- EXERCISE = child shows body movement during first 10 minutes of recess

REVIEW OF KCP SCHOOL PROCEDURES
- Nametags worn by children at lunch and recess (Monday, Wednesday, Friday)
- Token rewards given when children choose healthy be-haviors
- Reward days given weekly (Friday) to trade tokens for small prizes

---

KCP VOLUNTEER TASKS DURING LUNCH

- Stand near assigned lunch location (50 children if school lunch, 25 if home-packed)
- Note the time your assigned children begin eating
- Wait until 10 minutes later
- Punch one star in nametag for each healthy behavior (FV-FIRST, HDRINK)

KCP VOLUNTEER TASKS DURING RECESS

- Stand near location of recess (25–50 children, depending on size of playground)
- Note the time recess begins
- Wait until 10 minutes later
- Punch one star in nametag for body movement for the 10 minutes (EXERCISE)

KCP VOLUNTEER TASKS DURING REWARD DAY

- Volunteer #1
  o Count tokens (stars) in children's nametags
  o Mark nametags to "cancel" used tokens and show prizes earned
  o Call out number of smll prizes for each child
- Volunteer #2
  o Ask children to point to the plastic bin with prize(s) they choose
  o Hand children their chosen prize(s) from the plastic bins

Parent Records back to school on Reward Days, when each healthy behavior recorded at home earns them one additional token.

Another way in which parents can participate in the KCP goals to improve children's healthy behaviors is by including more fruits and vegetables and low-fat and low-sugar healthy drinks in home-packed lunches. We have documented that parents will include more healthy foods in their children's home-packed lunches when the KCP is being applied at their school, and their children respond with more healthy food choices of FVFIRST and HDRINK (Hendy et al., 2011).

TEXTBOX 5.2 PARENT RECORD OF HEALTHY BEHAVIORS AT HOME (OPTIONAL)

This 5-day record for the Kid's Choice Program (KCP) lets your child earn more Stars toward small prizes on Reward Day for healthy choices at home. Please send this record back to school with your child on Friday.

Child: _____ Parent signature: _____

Grade: _____ Teacher: _____

RECORD HEALTHY BEHAVIORS FOR FIVE DAYS (X = yes, O = no):

FVFIRST = child ate 1/8 cup FV in first 10 minutes of meal (about the size of a ping-pong ball)

HDRINK = child chose low-fat and low-sugar healthy drink (these can be skim or low-fat white milk, water, 100% juice, etc.)

EXERCISE = child showed body movement 10 minutes (these can be walking, running, climbing, soccer, basketball, etc.)

DATE	FVFIRST	HDRINK	EXERCISE
# DAYS BEHAVIOR SHOWN:			

Finally, parents may contribute to the KCP application at their children's school by serving as one of the volunteers who deliver the KCP three days each week (with one volunteer needed for each 50 children at lunch, and one volunteer needed for each 25–50 children at recess). As described in Chapter 4, we have documented that such small teams of 2–4 parent volunteers can effectively deliver the KCP three days per week, with children showing improvements in their FVFIRST, HDRINK, and EXERCISE behaviors (Hendy et al., 2011).

School leaders can encourage parent participation by including parent input in decisions about KCP procedures chosen for their children's school. For example, parents can help select which volunteers should deliver the KCP at their school (such as parents, grandparents, high school students, college students) and which types of small prizes will be made available on Reward Days (such as those shown in Chapter 5).

ENCOURAGING COMMUNITY INVOLVEMENT

During our own KCP applications, some of the fresh FV and prizes were donated by local businesses and organizations (e.g., toy stores, stationery stores, grocery stores, sporting goods stores, hospitals). With some creativity, parent-teacher organizations could also work with their own local businesses and organizations to reduce KCP costs and to provide environments outside school that also encourage children to choose healthy behaviors. Some examples would be maps of safe walking routes to school, special signs in grocery stores to help children identify healthy food choices, and lists of "exercise with friends" activities provided by sporting goods stores.

6

KCP APPLICATION: MATERIALS AND COSTS

KCP MATERIALS NEEDED

We designed the Kid's Choice Program (KCP) to be low in cost (at approximately US$2 per child per month of application) by using supplies already available in most elementary schools, with the exception of the small prizes used on Reward Day (Hendy et al., 2011). All the supplies needed for the KCP include:

- FVFIRST options available at lunch = 2+ choices of fruit and/ or vegetable
- HDRINK options available at lunch = 2+ choices of low-fat, low-sugar healthy drinks
- EXERCISE options available at recess = 2+ choices of body movement
- Nametag necklaces = using yarn and index cards (or laminated cards and lanyards)
- Token rewards = such as holes punched in nametags, stickers, plastic bracelets
- Small prizes for Reward Day = pencils, notebooks, puzzles, silly hats, school coupons

FVFIRST AND HDRINK OPTIONS AT LUNCH

Most school-provided lunches already provide one or two FV options that children can eat to accomplish the KCP healthy behavior of FVFIRST (eating 1/8 cup FV during the first 10 minutes of lunch). Even if potato foods are not counted (because they are typically prepared to be high in fat and salt), most school lunches would include another serving of canned, cooked, or fresh FV. For lunches that do not already provide two choices of FV, the second FV option can be provided with a large bowl of commonly available fresh FV such as apples, bananas, oranges, grapes, baby carrots, cherry tomatoes. (See Textbox 4.1 in Chapter 4 for a list of possible FV choices.)

Most school-provided lunches also provide 2+ drink options that allow children to accomplish the KCP healthy behavior of HDRINK (choosing low-fat and low-sugar healthy drinks). These drinks might include 1% or 2% white milk, skim milk, 100% fruit juice, or water. They would *not* include flavored milk drinks because they typically have added sugar, "fruit-flavored" drinks, or sodas of any kind including diet soda. (See Textbox 4.1 in Chapter 4 for a list of possible HDRINK choices.)

EXERCISE OPTIONS AT RECESS

Most schools provide recess facilities that offer children 2+ options for body movement to accomplish the third KCP health behavior of EXERCISE during the first 10 minutes of recess. Some examples of exercise activities would be playing basketball, playing soccer, jumping rope, having races, completing an obstacle course, climbing on playground structures, or simply walking. (See Textbox 4.1 in Chapter 4 for a list of possible EXERCISE choices.)

NAMETAG NECKLACES AND TOKEN REWARDS

The simplest nametag necklaces are made from supplies readily available in most schools. (See Textbox 6.1.) For example, index

---

TEXTBOX 6.1 INSTRUCTIONS FOR PREPARATION OF KCP NAMETAG NECKLACES

The nametag necklaces that are least expensive and easiest to prepare are made from supplies readily available in most schools. For example, index cards or other sturdy paper can be cut into shapes approximately 3 × 5 inches in dimension, with holes punched at one end, with string, yarn, or shoelaces of approximately 24 inches tied to these holes. Children can individualize their nametags with their names and drawings of their choice (such as the school's mascot). More durable and attractive nametag necklaces may be made with sturdy cover-weight paper in bright neon colors, with the whole paper laminated, then cut into sections approximately 3 × 5 inches in dimension, with holes punched at one end, and clipped to ½-inch-wide cloth lanyards printed with the name of the school. (See Photo 4.1.)

---

cards or other sturdy paper can be cut into shapes approximately 3 × 5 inches in dimensions, with holes punched at one end, with a piece of string or yarn of approximately 24 inches tied to these holes. Children can individualize their nametags with their names and drawings of their choice (such as the school's mascot). More durable and attractive nametags may be made with laminated cover-weight and neon-colored paper, clipped to ½-inch-wide cloth lanyards printed with the name of the school.

We use star-shaped holes punched into children's nametags as the token reward delivered immediately after children choose each KCP healthy behavior (FVFIRST, HDRINK, EXERCISE). These stars are attractive to children, and they allow us to describe to children the number of stars they need in exchange for each small prize on Reward Day. Other readily available and not easily altered tokens would be stickers applied to children's nametags, or a distinctive mark made with a colorful permanent pen. We have also used colorful plastic bracelets that children slip onto the strings of their nametag necklaces. (See Textbox 6.2.)

TEXTBOX 6.2 WHICH TOKEN REWARD FOR YOUR SCHOOL?

_____ star-shaped holes punched into nametags
_____ stickers on nametags
_____ distinctive marks written on nametags
_____ plastic rings or bracelets strung on nametag necklaces

TEXTBOX 6.3 WHICH SMALL PRIZES FOR YOUR SCHOOL?

_____ fancy pencils	_____ beach balls	_____ water bottles
_____ notebooks	_____ stuffed animals	_____ piggy banks
_____ puzzles	_____ silly hats	_____ bubble liquid
_____ pens	_____ playing cards	_____ collectible cards
_____ stickers	_____ small storage boxes	_____ jump ropes
_____ crayons	_____ modeling clay	_____ toy gliders

_____ coupons for special school privileges (first in lunch line, extra computer time, etc.)
_____ coupons donated for small items from toy stores
_____ coupons donated for small items from stationery stores
_____ coupons donated for small items from sporting goods stores
_____ coupons donated for small items from music stores
_____ coupons donated for small items from clothing stores
_____ coupons donated for small items from bookstores
_____ coupons donate for roller skating, bowling, miniature golf
_____ other _____

Note: Never use favorite sweets or snack foods as prizes! Research shows that children learn to like the sweets and snack foods *more*, while learning to like the healthy behaviors they had to do to earn them *less* (Newman & Taylor, 1992).

SMALL PRIZES FOR REWARD DAY

Some examples of inexpensive small prizes we use for Reward Day are puzzles, pens, modeling clay, fancy pencils, notebooks, piggy banks, toy gliders, books of stickers, water bottles, playing cards, jump ropes, stuffed animals, balls, and silly hats. (See Textbox 6.3.) These prizes usually cost 50 cents to $1 each when purchased in bulk from a variety of vendors. (See Textbox 6.4.) Coupons from school may also be used as prizes that give children valued privileges such as being first in the lunch line or having extra computer time. Coupons from local businesses could also be offered as prizes during Reward Day, such as those from the local stationery store for pens or notebooks, those from the local bowling alley or miniature golf course for free games, and those from the local sporting goods store for ping-pong balls, jump ropes, or pedometers.

SOURCES OF SUPPORT TO COVER KCP COSTS

School grants to support the cost of KCP supplies can come from a number of sources. These can include the state government, the federal government, nonprofit foundations, and corporations. (See Textbox 6.5.) Local fund-raisers could also be organized by the school's parent-teacher organization or by local high school or college students in education, health, nutrition, or child development classes.

TEXTBOX 6.4 WEBSITES OF POSSIBLE VENDORS FOR SMALL PRIZES

VENDOR	WEBSITE
COSTCO	www.costco.com
KMART	www.kmart.com
OFFICE DEPOT	www.officedepot.com
OFFICE MAX	www.officemax.com
RHODE ISLAND NOVELTY	www.rinovelty.com
SAM'S CLUB	www.samsclub.com
STAPLES	www.staples.com
TOYS R US	www.toysrus.com
WALMART	www.walmart.com

TEXTBOX 6.5 WEBSITES OF POSSIBLE GRANT SUPPORT FOR KCP SUPPLIES

ORGANIZATION	WEBSITE
Association of Schools of Public Health	www.asph.org
Center for Health and Health Care in Schools	www.healthinschools.org
Department of Agriculture	www.usda.gov
Department of Education	www.ed.gov
Department of Health and Human Services	www.hhs.gov
Food and Drug Administration	www.fda.gov
Gerber Foundation	www.gerberfoundation.org
Kellogg Foundation	www.wkkf.org
National Institutes of Health	www.nih.gov
National Science Foundation	www.nsf.gov

7

DOCUMENTING YOUR KCP EFFECTIVENESS (OPTIONAL)

W e have developed a few simple datasheets for use by school leaders (or health researchers) who wish to document their Kid's Choice Program's effectiveness for improving children's healthy behaviors, preferences for healthy behaviors, and weight status. We also have used a datasheet to rate KCP acceptability to school staff and parents, as well as to provide their suggestions for improvement. Such documentation can be valuable when a school requests funding support for of its KCP to improve children's healthy development.

DOCUMENTING CHANGES IN CHILDREN'S HEALTHY BEHAVIORS

To document changes in children's healthy behaviors at school lunch, we provide a datasheet that may be used by parent volunteers to record lunch behaviors during baseline conditions and KCP conditions. The two lunch behaviors recorded include eating FV first (FVFIRST) and choosing low-fat and low-sugar healthy drinks (HDRINK). (See Textbox 7.1.) To document changes in children's healthy behavior of EXERCISE at recess, we provide another datasheet that may be used by parent volunteers to record EXERCISE during baseline conditions and KCP conditions. (See Textbox 7.2.) Our experience suggests that the KCP increases children's FVFIRST, HDRINK, and EXERCISE behaviors as quickly as the first week it is implemented.

DOCUMENTING CHANGES IN CHILDREN'S PREFERENCES FOR FV

To document changes in children's preference ratings for FV (the food group most often rejected by picky eaters), we provide a child interview and datasheet that may be used by parent volunteers to record FV preferences during baseline conditions and after KCP application. (See Textbox 7.3.) To obtain a rating of KCP acceptability to children, one last question can be added to the child interview: "Please point to the face that shows me how much you liked the Kid's Choice Program provided at your school" (frowning face, "I don't like it" = 1; neutral face, "it's just OK" = 2; smiling face, "I like it" = 3). Our research shows that the KCP can significantly increase children's FV preference ratings after a one-month application, with high acceptability of the program by children (Hendy et al., 2005, 2011).

DOCUMENTING CHANGES IN CHILDREN'S WEIGHT STATUS

To document changes in children's BMI% weight status scores, we provide a datasheet that may be used by the school nurse to record children's BMI% scores during baseline conditions and after KCP application. (See Textbox 7.4.) Our research shows that the KCP can significantly decrease BMI% scores for overweight children after a three-month application, as well as maintaining healthy BMI% scores for normal-weight children (Hendy et al., 2011).

DOCUMENTING KCP ACCEPTABILITY FOR SCHOOL STAFF AND PARENTS

To document the acceptability of various KCP procedures for school staff and parents, we provide a brief survey that may be used by school leaders to determine which KCP options would work best at their schools. (See Textbox 7.5.) Our research suggests that highest acceptability ratings are given to the KCP procedures of nametags worn by children at lunch and recess, star-shaped holes punched into nametags as the immediate token reward, Reward Days presented once weekly, optional Parent Records used to report children's healthy behaviors at home, and parent volunteers used to deliver the KCP. Least acceptable KCP options were the use of pedometers to record EXERCISE (because children often forgot, lost, or broke them), and the use of busy school staff to deliver the program (Hendy et al., 2011).

Additionally, school staff and parents may appreciate having input into other details of the KCP application given at their school. To gather their ideas, school leaders could ask their opinions about which specific FVFIRST, HDRINK, and EXERCISE options should be offered to the children during lunch and recess (as in Textbox 4.1), which token reward system should be used (as in Textbox 6.2), or which small prizes should be offered during Reward Days (as in Textbox 6.3).

TEXTBOX 7.1 DATASHEET TO RECORD FVFIRST AND HDRINK AT LUNCH

Note: This datasheet can be used under baseline conditions *before* the KCP application, then *after* the KCP application to examine changes in children's behavior.

Grade: _____ Teacher:_____

Study phase (baseline, KCP): _____

PLACE X IN THE BOX IF CHILD SHOWS FVFIRST (FV) OR HDRINK (HD) AT LUNCH:

	MON		WED		FRI		MON		WED		FRI			
CHILD	FV	HD	FV	HD	FV	HD	FV	HD	FV	HD	FV	HD	FV TOTAL	HD TOTAL

TEXTBOX 7.2 DATASHEET TO RECORD EXERCISE AT RECESS

Note: This datasheet can be used under baseline conditions *before* the KCP application, then *after* the KCP application to examine changes in children's behavior.

Grade: _____ Teacher: _____

Study phase (baseline, KCP): _____

PLACE X IN THE BOX IF CHILD SHOWS
EXERCISE DURING FIRST 10 MINUTES OF RECESS

CHILD	MON	WED	FRI	MON	WED	FRI	EXERCISE TOTAL

TEXTBOX 7.3 CHILD INTERVIEW FOR FV PREFERENCE RATINGS

Note: This datasheet can be used under baseline conditions *before* the KCP application, then *after* the KCP application to examine changes in children's preference ratings for FV.

Grade: _____ Teacher: _____

Study phase (baseline, KCP): _____

SCRIPT: Hello, my name is X. I came to your school to ask children how much they like different kinds of foods.

Let's use the three faces on this card to make it easier—

    Which face do we use to show we don't like

    something?   (FROWNING FACE = 1)

    Which face do we use to show that something

    is just OK?   (NEUTRAL FACE = 2)

    Which face do we use to show we really like

    something?   (SMILING FACE = 3)

Now, please point to the face that shows how much you like each food.

CHILD	pear	green beans	apple	tomato	peach	carrot	pine-apple	celery	banana	peas	MEAN = SUM / 10

TEXTBOX 7.4 DATASHEET TO RECORD CHILDREN'S WEIGHT CHANGE

Note: This datasheet can be used by the school nurse under baseline conditions *before* the KCP application, then *after* the KCP application to examine changes in children's weight status as measured by their body mass index percentile score (BMI%).

Grade: _____ Teacher: _____

WRITE EACH CHILD'S BMI% SCORE IN THE BOX FOR EACH STUDY PHASE

CHILD	Baseline BMI%	KCP (3 months) BMI%	KCP (6 months) BMI%

TEXTBOX 7.5 DATASHEET FOR STAFF AND PARENT FEEDBACK ON KCP

Please give us your opinions!

The Kid's Choice Program (KCP) we have been using at our school was designed as a school-based program to improve children's healthy behaviors, their preferences for these healthy behaviors, and their healthy weight status. The three healthy behaviors targeted include:

(1) FVFIRST = eat FV in the first 10 minutes of meals when hungry and when foods taste best

(2) HDRINK = choose a low-fat and low-sugar healthy drink for meals

(3) EXERCISE = show body movement in the first 10 minutes of recess.

The KCP uses simple school procedures:

(1) Children wear nametag necklaces three days a week at lunch and recess

(2) Children get small token rewards ("stars" on nametags) if they choose healthy behaviors

(3) Children can trade tokens for small prizes at a weekly Reward Day

(4) Small teams of 2–4 volunteers can deliver the KCP at lunch and recess

Research suggests that the KCP is effective because it includes the following components:

(1) 2+ choices available for each healthy behavior

(2) Small repeated experiences for each healthy behavior

(3) Small token rewards as incentives to try healthy behaviors

(4) Many peer models to demonstrate healthy behaviors

Before we continue the KCP at our school, we would like your feedback on how much you support each KCP option. Your input will help guide us to improve the KCP so that it can be a user-friendly and cost-effective program to improve the health of children at our school.

KCP FEEDBACK FROM SCHOOL STAFF AND PARENTS

(Please return to your child's teacher or the front office.)

_____ What is your role at our school? (1 = school staff, 2 = parent, 3 = both)

Please rate your opinion about the acceptability of each KCP option described below. Use a 5-point rating of acceptability (from 1 = not at all to 5 = very much).

_____ Children wear nametags at school lunch

_____ Children wear nametags at school recess

_____ "Stars" on nametags (or other token rewards) given to children for healthy choices

_____ Reward Days are held weekly so children can trade "stars" (tokens) for small prizes

_____ Pedometers are worn by children to record their exercise

_____ Recess checklists (rather than pedometers) are used to record children's exercise

_____ "Parent Records" are used to record children's healthy behaviors at home

_____ KCP lunch and recess observations and Reward Day are delivered by school staff

_____ KCP lunch and recess observations and Reward Day are delivered by PTO volunteers

_____ KCP lunch and recess observations and Reward Day delivered by older children

_____ KCP lunch and recess observations and Reward Day delivered by local college students

_____ Please rate the overall acceptability of the Kid's Choice Program used at our school

WHAT ARE THE MOST EFFECTIVE KCP FEATURES?

WHAT ARE KCP FEATURES NEEDING IMPROVEMENT?

8

OTHER PARENT MEALTIME ACTIONS

Chapter 5 included descriptions of how parents could participate in the school-based Kid's Choice Program to make it a true "school-home partnership" for encouraging children's healthy behaviors and reducing the risk of child obesity. For example, parents could complete weekly Parent Records of their children's healthy behaviors (FVFIRST, HDRINK, EXERCISE) at home so that children could receive additional token rewards ("stars") toward earning small prizes on the weekly Reward Days. Parents could also participate as KCP volunteers to deliver stars to children's nametags during school lunch and recess when they choose healthy behaviors or to deliver the weekly Reward Days when children trade tokens for small prizes.

The present chapter describes other research-backed actions that parents can do at home to encourage their children to develop a healthy diet and weight status. It is well known that children and their parents influence each other during family meals (Ventura & Birch, 2008), but Costanzo and Woody (1985) suggested that certain parent feeding practices might influence children's ability to learn "self-regulation" of their food intake. Since then, a number of researchers have conducted studies to identify which specific parent feeding practices are most associated with children's diet and weight status (and for reviews, see Faith et al., 2004; Savage et al., 2007; Wardle & Carnell, 2006).

PARENT MEALTIME ACTIONS ASSOCIATED WITH CHILDREN'S DIET AND WEIGHT

Research suggests that when parents model healthy eating habits such as eating many FV and few snack foods, their children are more likely to develop similar eating habits (Hendy, Williams, Camise, Eckman, et al., 2009). Additionally, when parents calmly set mealtime expectations that children "try one bite" of the foods included in shared family meals, their children are more likely to eat many daily servings of FV, perhaps because these small "bites" gradually help children reach the threshold of 8–10 small-taste experiences they may need to learn to "like" new foods (Birch et al., 1987; Wardle et al., 2003).

Other parent actions appear to be *in response* to children's weight, mealtime behavior, or other characteristics. For example, parents respond to news that their child is overweight by using less pressure to eat during meals and by restricting fat consumption (Faith et al., 2004; Grimmett et al., 2008; Hendy, Williams, Camise, Eckman, et al., 2009; Hendy & Williams, 2012; Kroller & Warschburger, 2008; Sanders et al., 1993; Spruijt-Metz et al., 2002; Webber et al., 2010). Unfortunately, forbidding children to eat their favorite foods tends to backfire and result in overconsumption of these foods when children have the opportunity (Baughcum et al., 2001; Fisher & Birch, 1999).

While forbidding children to eat foods that are already in the home may be counterproductive (e.g., "your brother can have cookies because he is not fat like you"), an alternative approach is parental control of the food that enters the home in the first place. For example, research has shown that the availability of FV at home is associated with children eating more of these healthy foods (Cullen et al., 2003; Hendy, Williams, Camise, Eckman et al., 2009). It is important that parents understand that healthy eating starts at the *point of purchase* so that children's exposure is primarily to healthy items.

Parents appear to respond to children's picky eating by using enthusiastic persuasion then by giving up and using nutritional supplements or preparing "special meals" for their picky eaters that are different from the shared family meal (Hendy, Williams, Camise, Eckman et al., 2009; Hendy et al., 2010; Hughes et al., 2008; Lockner et al., 2008; Schreck et al., 2004). Parents often turn to such "special meals" when concerned that their children are underweight or to avoid disruptive behavior during meals (Rhoe et al., 2006). However, research suggests that although such "special meals" may reduce the child's risk of being underweight, they also may prevent children from ever learning to eat a healthy variety of foods (Hendy et al., 2010; Seiverling et al., 2011).

Other demographic characteristics have been found associated with parent feeding practices. Mothers are more likely than fathers to be the "nutrition gatekeepers" for their children with the purchase, preparation, and serving of foods (McIntosh & Zey, 1989). Mothers tend to give more guidance in food selection to younger than older children (Hendy & Williams, 2012; Savage et al., 2007), and they report more concern about overweight in daughters than sons (Maynard et al., 2003). Children living in poverty have more risk for overweight (Darmon & Drewnowski, 2008; Hendy & Williams, 2012), perhaps because parents cannot afford healthy food options, have less education about nutrition, or must focus more on avoiding hunger than avoiding overweight. (Please see Textbox 8.1 for suggested readings on parent mealtime actions.)

MEASURING PARENT MEALTIME ACTIONS

The Parent Mealtime Action Scale (PMAS) was developed as a research, clinical, and educational tool to help identify patterns of parent feeding practices (Hendy et al., 2009). The PMAS has been validated with samples of nearly 3,000 children sampled from preschools and elementary schools, as with samples of more than 200 children sampled from a hospital-based feeding clinic (Hendy et al., 2009; Williams et al., 2011). Nine dimensions of parent mealtime action were identified:

TEXTBOX 8.1 READINGS ON PARENT MEALTIME ACTIONS

Fisher, J. O., & Birch, L. L. (1999). Restricting access to foods and children's eating. *Appetite, 32,* 405–419.

Grimmett, C., Croker, H., Carnell, S., & Wardle, J. (2008). Telling parents their child's weight status: Psychological impact of a weight-screening program. *Pediatrics, 122,* 682–688.

Hendy, H. M., & Williams, K. E. (2012). Mother's feeding practices for children 3 to 10 years of age and their associations with child demographics. *Appetite, 58,* 710–716.

Hendy, H. M., Williams, K. E., Camise, T. S., Eckman, N., & Hedemann, A. (2009). The Parent Mealtime Action Scale (PMAS): Development and association with children's diet and weight. *Appetite, 52,* 328–339.

Hendy, H. M., Williams, K. E., Riegel, K., & Paul, C. (2010). Parent mealtime actions that mediate associations between children's fussy eating and their weight and diet. *Appetite, 54,* 191–195.

- Snack limits = parent sets limits on the child's snack foods high in fat, sugar, salt
- Positive persuasion = parent enthusiastically says how good foods taste
- Daily FV availability = parent eats and serves the child FV daily
- Use of rewards = parent offers favorite foods or special activities for eating foods
- Insistence on eating = parent sets mealtime expectations for small tastes
- Snack modeling = parent eats snack foods high in fat, sugar, salt
- Special meals = parent prepares child special meals, different from family meal
- Fat reduction = parent serves child low-fat versions of foods
- Many food choices = parent allows child to eat whatever he/she wants

Please see Textbox 8.2 for the Parent Mealtime Action Scale (PMAS), Textbox 8.3 for instructions for scoring the nine PMAS dimensions, and Textbox 8.4 for norms for samples of average-developing and feeding-clinic children. For translations of the PMAS, please see Textbox 8.5 for Chinese, Textbox 8.6 for Farsi, Textbox 8.7 for French, Textbox 8.8 for German, Textbox 8.9 for Korean, Textbox 8.10 for Portuguese, Textbox 8.11 for Spanish, and Textbox 8.12 for Turkish. (For additional translations of the PMAS, please contact Dr. Helen Hendy at hl4@psu.edu.)

RECOMMENDED PARENT MEALTIME ACTIONS

Our research has documented that some parent feeding practices measured by the PMAS are significantly associated with children's healthy diet and weight status (Hendy, Williams, Camise, Eckman et al., 2010, 2012; Williams, Hendy, and Knecht, 2008; Williams et al., 2011). Based on research results, we recommend two mealtime actions that parents should *do* and three that they should *avoid*:

DO
- o Positive persuasion = parent enthusiastically says how good foods taste
- o Daily FV availability = parent eats and serves the child FV daily

AVOID
- o Snack modeling = parent eats snack foods high in fat, sugar, salt
- o Special meals = parent prepares child special meals, different from family meal
- o Many food choices = parent allows child to eat whatever he/she wants

TEXTBOX 8.2 THE PARENT MEALTIME ACTION SCALE (PMAS)

During a typical week, how often do you show each mealtime action?
Please circle the appropriate number.

Parent Mealtime Actions	1 = never 2 = sometimes 3 = always
1. You made eating the food a game or fun for the child	1 2 3
2. You ate the same foods as those offered to the child	1 2 3
3. You sat with the child, but did not eat	1 2 3
4. You let the child eat whatever he/she wanted	1 2 3
5. You let the child flavor the food however he/she wanted	1 2 3
6. You gave the child a favorite food as a reward for good behavior	1 2 3
7. You offered the child a toy or favorite activity as a reward for eating	1 2 3
8. You offered the child a special dessert as a reward for eating	1 2 3
9. You let the child substitute a food for one he/she liked	1 2 3
10. You let the child choose foods to eat, but only from those offered	1 2 3
11. You prepared a special meal for the child, different from family meal	1 2 3
12. You stopped the child from eating too much	1 2 3
13. You told the child how much you liked the food	1 2 3
14. You told the child how good the food will taste if he/she tries it	1 2 3
15. You told the child that his/her friends or siblings like the food	1 2 3
16. You told the child that a food will make him/her healthy, smart, strong	1 2 3
17. You gave the child fruit each day	1 2 3
18. You made changes to the child's food to lower fat	1 2 3
19. You ate fruit each day	1 2 3
20. You ate vegetables each day	1 2 3
21. You drank soda each day	1 2 3
22. You ate candy or sweets each day	1 2 3
23. You ate salty snacks each day	1 2 3
24. You made changes to your own food to lower fat	1 2 3
25. You set limits for how many sweets the child could have each day	1 2 3
26. You set limits for how many sodas the child could have each day	1 2 3
27. You set limits for how many salty snacks the child could have each day	1 2 3
28. You insisted the child eat even if he/she said "I'm not hungry"	1 2 3
29. You insisted the child eat when he/she was sleepy, not feeling well	1 2 3
30. You insisted the child eat when he/she was emotionally upset	1 2 3
31. You placed some of each food on the child's plate	1 2 3

TEXTBOX 8.3 SCORING NINE PMAS DIMENSIONS

Steps:
   (1) For each PMAS dimension, record ratings for all items in the dimension.
   (2) Sum all ratings in the dimension.
   (3) Divide the sum by the number of items in the dimension.

SNACK LIMITS:
   Ratings: ____ + ____ + ____ = _____ (Sum)
   Item #:   25   26   27
   Snack limits score is this sum divided by 3 = _____

POSITIVE PERSUASION:
   Ratings: ____ + ____ + ____ + ____ = _____ (Sum)
   Item #:   13   14   15   16
   Positive persuasion score is this sum divided by 4 = _____

DAILY FV AVAILABILITY:
   Ratings: ____ + ____ + ____ = _____ (Sum)
   Item #:   17   19   20
   Daily FV availability score is this sum divided by 3 = _____

USE OF REWARDS:
   Ratings: ____ + ____ + ____ + ____ = _____ (Sum)
   Item #:   1   6   7   8
   Use of rewards score is this sum divided by 4 = _____

INSISTENCE ON EATING:
   Ratings: ____ + ____ + ____ = _____ (Sum)
   Item #:   28   29   30
   Insistence on eating score is this sum divided by 3 = ____

SNACK MODELING:
   Ratings: ____ + ____ + ____ = _____ (Sum)
   Item #:   21   22   23
   Snack modeling score is this sum divided by 3 = _____

SPECIAL MEALS:
First, reverse the ratings given for Item 2 and Item 31 (only) so that 1 = 3, 2 = 2, 3 = 1.
(new) Ratings: ____ + ____ + ____ + ____ = _____ (Sum)
Item #:   2   3   11   31
Special meals score is this sum divided by 4 = _____

FAT REDUCTION:
Ratings: ____ + ____ + ____ = _____ (Sum)
Item #:   12   18   24
Fat reduction score is this sum divided by 3 = _____

MANY FOOD CHOICES:
Ratings: ____ + ____ + ____ + ____ = _____ (Sum)
Item #:   4   5   9   10
Many food choices score is this sum divided by 4 = _____

TEXTBOX 8.4 NORMS FOR NINE PMAS DIMENSIONS

Note: Values shown are mean three-point ratings for parent action (1 = never, 2 = sometimes, 3 = always).

	Preschool age		School age	
	Average-developing children (n = 97)	Feeding-clinic children (n = 147)	Average-developing children (n = 2008)	Feeding-clinic children (n = 64)
PMAS DIMENSION	MEAN (SD)	MEAN (SD)	MEAN (SD)	MEAN (SD)
Snack Limits	2.65 (.51)	2.00 (.78)	2.60 (.51)	2.15 (.69)
Positive Persuasion	2.28 (.43)	2.24 (.56)	2.05 (.43)	2.36 (.53)
Daily FV Availability	2.45 (.45)	2.46 (.44)	2.45 (.43)	2.31 (.42)
Use of Rewards	1.84 (.38)	1.65 (.46)	1.49 (.35)	1.77 (.41)
Insistence on Eating	1.38 (.48)	1.33 (.45)	1.34 (.37)	1.34 (.37)
Snack Modeling	1.98 (.51)	1.82 (.43)	1.92 (.41)	1.82 (.42)
Special Meals	1.83 (.26)	1.96 (.42)	1.45 (.33)	1.78 (.41)
Fat Reduction	1.64 (.52)	1.41 (.34)	1.86 (.49)	1.53 (.49)
Many Food Choices	1.87 (.30)	1.91 (.49)	1.98 (.33)	2.15 (.45)

TEXTBOX 8.5 CHINESE TRANSLATION OF PMAS

Provided by Ping Wang, Ph.D.
Professor of Mathematics
Penn State University
Schuylkill Campus, PA

在过去一月随便一周里，你如何进行如下的事项的?
请在每项后选适当的答案.

家长餐时操作	1 = 从不 2 = 有时 3 = 总是		
1. 让吃东西成有趣的活动或游戏	1	2	3
2. 吃给孩子同样的食物	1	2	3
3. 坐观孩子吃	1	2	3
4. 让孩子决定吃什么	1	2	3
5. 让孩子决定食物的味道	1	2	3
6. 给孩子喜爱的食物作为平时的奖励	1	2	3
7. 给孩子玩具等作为吃东西的奖励	1	2	3
8. 给孩子甜点作为吃东西的奖励	1	2	3
9. 让孩子替换他不喜欢的食物	1	2	3
10. 让孩子选择食物	1	2	3
11. 为孩子准备专门的实物	1	2	3
12. 不让孩子吃过多	1	2	3
13. 告诉孩子你多么喜欢这食物	1	2	3
14. 告诉孩子如果他尝尝后会知道食物味道很不错	1	2	3
15. 告诉孩子他的姐弟朋友都喜欢这食物	1	2	3
16. 告诉孩子这食物会使他变得更健康，聪明，强壮	1	2	3
17. 每天给小孩水果	1	2	3
18. 给孩子低脂肪食物	1	2	3
19. 你自己天天吃水果	1	2	3
20. 你自己天天吃蔬菜	1	2	3
21. 你天天喝（含糖）饮料	1	2	3
22. 你天天吃甜点，糖果	1	2	3
23. 你天天吃咸饼干	1	2	3
24. 你自己减少食物里的脂肪	1	2	3
25. 规定小孩吃甜点的限度	1	2	3
26. 规定小孩每天喝（含糖）饮料的限度	1	2	3
27. 规定小孩每天吃咸饼干的限度	1	2	3
28. 小孩称"不饿"时，也坚持让他吃东西	1	2	3
29. 小孩发困，不舒服时，也坚持让他吃东西	1	2	3
30. 小孩情绪不好时，也坚持让他吃东西	1	2	3
31. 每次给小孩一些餐桌上各种不同的食物	1	2	3

TEXTBOX 8.6 FARSI TRANSLATION OF PMAS

Provided by Mohammad Rezaei, M.S.

Professor of Rehabilitation Sciences, Iran

and

Farideh Bowman

Schuylkill Haven, PA

مقیاس عملکرد والدین در حین غذا خوردن

هر یک از عملکردهای زیر را در حین غذا خوردن به چه میزان نشان دادهاید(در طول یک هفته از ماه گذشته)؟
لطفاً دور عدد مناسب خط بکشید.

1 : هرگز 2: برخی اوقات 3 : همیشه	عملکردهای والدین در حین صرف غذا
3 2 1	1. غذا خوردن را برای کودک به صورت بازی یا سرگرمی ایجاد میکنید؟
3 2 1	2. همان غذاهایی را میخورید که به کودک پیشنهاد میدهید؟
3 2 1	3. با کودکان مینشینید ولی غذا نمیخورید؟
3 2 1	4. به کودک اجازه میدهید هر چه میخواهد بخورد؟
3 2 1	5. به کودک اجازه میدهید غذا را به هر صورت که میخواهد مزمزه کند؟
3 2 1	6. به کودکتان غذای مورد علاقهاش را به عنوان پاداش برای غذا خوردن میدهید؟
3 2 1	7. به کودکتان فعالیت مورد علاقه یا اسباب بازی به عنوان پاداش برای غذا خوردن میدهید؟
3 2 1	8. به کودک اجازه میدهید غذایش را با غذای مورد علاقهاش جابجا کند؟
3 2 1	9. به کودکتان یک دسر مخصوص به عنوان پاداش برای غذا خوردن میدهید؟
3 2 1	10. به کودک اجازه میدهید از میان غذاهایی که شما پیشنهاد کردهاید، خودش نوع غذا را انتخاب کند؟
3 2 1	11. یک وعده غذایی مخصوص، متفاوت از وعده غذایی خانواده برای کودک فراهم میکنید؟
3 2 1	12. کودک را از زیاد خوردن منع میکنید؟
3 2 1	13. به کودک میگویید که خودتان غذا را چه مقدار دوست دارید؟
3 2 1	14. به کودکان میگویید اگر غذا را امتحان(مزه) کند، خوشمزه خواهد بود؟
3 2 1	15. به کودک میگویید که دوستان، خواهر و برادرانش غذا را دوست دارند؟
3 2 1	16. به کودک میگویید که غذا او را قوی، باهوش و سلامت نگه میدارد؟
3 2 1	17. هر روز به کودک میوه میدهید؟
3 2 1	18. آیا به منظور کاهش چربی در غذای کودک تغییر ایجاد میکنید ؟
3 2 1	19. روزانه میوه میخورید؟
3 2 1	20. روزانه سبزیجات میخورید؟
3 2 1	21. روزانه نوشیدنی(نوشابه و دلستر) میخورید؟
3 2 1	22. روزانه شیرینی و شکلات میخورید؟
3 2 1	23. روزانه میان وعده های شور(مانند پفک) میخورید؟
3 2 1	24. آیا به منظور کاهش چربی در غذای خودتان تغییر ایجاد میکنید؟
3 2 1	25. محدودیتی برای میزان شیرینی که کودک میتواند در طول روز بخورد، ایجاد میکنید؟
3 2 1	26. محدودیتی برای میزان نوشیدنی که کودک میتواند در طول روز بنوشد، ایجاد میکنید؟
3 2 1	27. برای مقدار میان وعده های شور کودک در طول روز، محدودیت ایجاد میکنید؟
3 2 1	28. حتی اگر کودکتان بگوید "من گرسنه نیستم" برای غذا خوردن پافشاری میکنید؟
3 2 1	29. آیا هنگامی که کودکتان خواب آلود بوده و احساس خوبی نداشته باشد، برای غذا خوردن پافشاری میکنید؟
3 2 1	30. آیا وقتی کودکتان آشفتگی روانی(مانند بیقراری و بیحوصلگی) دارد، باز هم برای غذا خوردن پافشاری میکنید؟
3 2 1	31. آیا مقداری از هر نوع غذا در بشقاب کودکتان قرار میدهید؟

TEXTBOX 8.7 FRENCH TRANSLATION OF PMAS

Provided by Sunbul Rai, M.S.

Autism Services

Saskatoon, Saskatchewan

Canada

Pendant une semaine typique, combien de fois montrez-vous à chacun l'action de repas?

Veuillez encercler le numéro approprie après chaque action.

Actions de repas des parents	1 = Jamais 2 = Parfois 3 = Toujours		
1. Vous avez fait manger la nourriture un jeu ou un amusement pour l'enfant	1	2	3
2. Vous avez mangé la même alimentation que votre enfant	1	2	3
3. Vous vous êtes assis avec l'enfant mais n'avais pas mangez	1	2	3
4. Vous aves laissez l'enfant manger ce qu'il/elle veut	1	2	3
5. Vous laissez l'enfant gouter son repas comme qu'il/elle veuille	1	2	3
6. Vous avez donné l'enfant son repas préféré pour récompenser sa bonne conduite	1	2	3
7. Vous offrez l'enfant son jeu préféré ou son activité préférer en récompense pour avoir mangé	1	2	3
8. Vous avez offert à l'enfant un dessert spécial comme récompense pour avoir mangé	1	2	3
9. Vous laisser l'enfant substituer un aliment qu'il/elle aime	1	2	3
10. Vous laissez l'enfant a choisir l'aliment a manger parmi ceux offert	1	2	3
11. Vous avez préparé un repas spéciale pour l'enfant qui est différent du repas familiale	1	2	3
12. Vous avez prévenu l'enfant de trop manger	1	2	3
13. Vous dites a l'enfant combien vous aimez le repas	1	2	3
14. Vous avez dit a l'enfant combine le repas goutera bon s'il/elle essaye	1	2	3
15. Vous dites a l'enfant que son frère, sœur et ami aime le repas	1	2	3
16. Vous avez dit a l'enfant que l'aliment lui apportera de la santé, futée et va lui faire fort	1	2	3
17. Vous avez donné des fruits à l'enfant a chaque jour	1	2	3
18. Vous avez apporté des changements à l'alimentation de l'enfant pour abaisser le gras	1	2	3
19. Vous avez consommé des fruits à chaque jour	1	2	3
20. Vous avez consommé des légumes à chaque jour	1	2	3
21. Vous avez bu des boissons gazeuses chaque jour	1	2	3
22. Vous avez consommé des bonbons ou des sucreries chaque jour	1	2	3
23. Vous avez consommé des collations salées chaque jour	1	2	3
24. Vous avez apporte des changements a votre alimentation pour abaisser le gras	1	2	3
25. Vous limiter le nombre de sucreries que l'enfant peut avoir chaque jour	1	2	3
26. Vous limiter le nombre de boissons gazeuses que l'enfant peut avoir chaque jour	1	2	3
27. Vous limiter le nombre de collations salées que l'enfant peut avoir chaque jour	1	2	3
28. Vous insister que l'enfant mange lorsqu'il/elle dit "Je n'ai pas faim"	1	2	3
29. Vous insister que l'enfant mange lorsqu'il/elle se sent endormi ou mal a l'aise	1	2	3
30. Vous insister l'enfant de manger lorsqu'il/elle se sent bouleverser	1	2	3
31. Vous placer un peu de chaque aliment dans le plat de l'enfant	1	2	3

TEXTBOX 8.8 GERMAN TRANSLATION OF PMAS

Provided by Hartmut Heep, Ph.D.

Associate Professor of Languages and Comparative Literature

Penn State University

Schuylkill Campus, PA

Wie oft zeigten Sie die folgenden Verhaltensformen bei den Mahlzeiten während einer typischen Woche des letzten Monats. Bieten kreisen Sie die entsprechende Zahl ein.

Eltern Mahlzeit Handungen	1 = niemals 2 = manchmal 3 = immer
1. Die Mahlzeit wurde zur positive Spielzeit für das Kind	1 2 3
2. Sie aßen dasselbe Gericht wie Ihr Kind	1 2 3
3. Sie saßen mit dem Kind, ohne selbst zu essen	1 2 3
4. Das Kind durfte essen, was es wollte	1 2 3
5. Das Kind durfte sein Essen selbst würzen	1 2 3
6. Das Kind bekam ein Lieblingsgericht zur Belohnung	1 2 3
7. Das Kind bekam ein Spielzeug oder Lieblingsaktivität zur Belohnung	1 2 3
8. Das Kind bekam einen besonderen Nachtisch zur Belohnung	1 2 3
9. Das Kind durfte einen Teil der Mahlzeit mit einem Lieblingsnahrungsmittel ersetzen	1 2 3
10. Das Kind konnte aus einer begrenzten Auswahl sein Menu selbst zusammenstellen	1 2 3
11. Das Kind bekam eine besondere Mahlzeit, anders als der Rest der Familie	1 2 3
12. Sie stoppten das Kind vom Zuvielessen	1 2 3
13. Sie sagten dem Kind wie sehr Sie das Essen mögen	1 2 3
14. Sie sagten dem Kind wie lecker das Essen sei, wenn es es nur mal probiere	1 2 3
15. Sie sagten dem Kind, dass seine Freunde/ Geschwister das Essen mögen	1 2 3
16. Sie sagten dem Kind, dass man vom Essen gesund, intelligent, und stark wer	1 2 3
17. Sie gaben dem Kind jeden Tag Obst	1 2 3
18. Sie bereiteten die Mahlzeit des Kindes fettarmer	1 2 3
19. Sie aßen täglich Obst	1 2 3
20. Sie aßen täglich Gemüse	1 2 3
21. Sie tranken täglich Getränke mit Kohlensäure	1 2 3
22. Sie aßen täglich Süßigkeiten	1 2 3
23. Sie aßen täglich salziges Gebäck	1 2 3
24. Sie stellten ihre eigene Mahlzeit auf fettarm um	1 2 3
25. Dem Kind wurde nur eine begrenzte Anzahl von Süßigkeiten geben	1 2 3
26. Dem Kind wurde nur eine begrenzte Anzahl von Getränken mit Kohlensäure gegeben	1 2 3
27. Dem Kind wurde nur eine begrenzte Anzahl von salzigem Gebäck gegeben	1 2 3
28. Sie zwangen das Kind zum Essen, selbst wenn es nicht hungrig war	1 2 3
29. Sie zwangen das Kind zum Essen, selbst wenn es müde/krank war	1 2 3
30. Sie zwangen das Kind zum Essen, selbst wenn es aufgeregt war	1 2 3
31. Sie gaben dem Kind das Essen auf seinen Teller	1 2 3

TEXTBOX 8.9 KOREAN TRANSLATION OF PMAS

Provided by Kyong-Mee Chung, Ph.D.
and
Jeong Hyun Choo, Ph.D.
Department of Psychology
Yonsei University, Seoul, Korea

보통 한 주 동안 다음과 같은 행동을 얼마나 하십니까? 각 문항에 대해 적절한 숫자로 표시하여 주십시오.

부모의 식사시간 행동	1 = 전혀 2 = 때때로 3 = 항상		
1. 아이를 위해 음식 먹는 것을 게임이나 재미있는 놀이로 만들었다	1	2	3
2. 아이에게 준 음식과 같은 것을 나도 먹었다	1	2	3
3. 아이와 함께 식사 자리에 앉긴 했지만 나는 먹지 않았다	1	2	3
4. 아이가 원하는 음식은 어떤 것이든 먹게 해주었다	1	2	3
5. 아이가 원하는 대로 음식의 맛을 바꿀 수 있게 허락해 주었다	1	2	3
6. 잘한 행동에 대한 보상으로 아이가 가장 좋아하는 음식을 주었다	1	2	3
7. 먹는 것에 대한 보상으로 아이에게 장난감을 주거나 아이가 가장 좋아하는 활동을 하게 해 주었다	1	2	3
8. 먹는 것에 대한 보상으로 아이에게 특별한 디저트를 주었다	1	2	3
9. 아이가 좋아하는 음식으로 바꿔먹는 것을 허락했다	1	2	3
10. 차린 음식들 중에서 아이 자신이 먹을 음식을 선택하게 해주었다	1	2	3
11. 아이를 위해 가족과는 다른 특별한 식사를 준비하였다	1	2	3
12. 아이가 너무 많이 먹지 못하게 하였다	1	2	3
13. 내가 특정 음식에 대해 얼마나 좋아했는지 아이에게 말해주었다	1	2	3
14. 음식을 맛보면 얼마나 그 맛이 맛날 지 아이에게 알려주었다	1	2	3
15. 아이의 친구 또는 형제들이 그 음식을 좋아한다고 아이에게 말해주었다	1	2	3
16. 아이에게 특정 음식이 건강하고, 똑똑하고, 힘세게 만들어 줄 것이라고 말해주었다	1	2	3
17. 아이에게 매일 과일을 주었다	1	2	3
18. 아이에게 줄 음식을 저지방식으로 바꿨다	1	2	3
19. 나는 매일 과일을 먹었다	1	2	3
20. 나는 매일 채소를 먹었다	1	2	3
21. 나는 매일 탄산음료를 마셨다	1	2	3
22. 나는 매일 사탕이나 단 음식을 먹었다	1	2	3
23. 나는 매일 짠 간식을 먹었다	1	2	3
24. 내가 먹는 음식을 저지방식으로 바꿨다	1	2	3
25. 아이가 하루에 먹을 수 있는 단 음식의 을 제한하였다	1	2	3
26. 아이가 하루에 마실 수 있는 탄산음료의 양을 제한하였다	1	2	3
27. 아이가 하루에 먹을 수 있는 짠 음식의 양을 제한하였다	1	2	3
28. 아이가 "배고프지 않아"라고 말했을 경우에도 먹으라고 하였다	1	2	3
29. 아이가 졸릴 때나 몸 상태가 별로 좋지 않을 때도 먹으라고 하였다	1	2	3
30. 아이가 속이 상해 있을 때도 먹으라고 하였다	1	2	3
31. 아이가 식사할 때 접시에 각각의 음식을 조금씩 놓아주었다	1	2	3

TEXTBOX 8.10 PORTUGUESE TRANSLATION OF PMAS

Provided by Maria Luiza Petty, M.A.

Department of Nutrition

Federal University of Sao Paulo, Brazil

Durante uma semana típica, com que freqüência você exibe cada um dos seguintes comportamentos?

COMPORTAMENTO DOS PAIS DURANTE AS REFEIÇÕES	1 - NUNCA 2 - ÀS VEZES 3 - SEMPRE
1. Você faz com que o momento de comer seja um jogo ou uma diverção para a criança	1 2 3
2. Você come os mesmos alimentos que são oferecidos para a criança	1 2 3
3. Você se senta com a criança, mas não come	1 2 3
4. Você deixa a criança comer o que ela quiser	1 2 3
5. Você deixa a criança colocar temperos/molhos na comida como ela quer	1 2 3
6. Você dá para a criança um alimento preferido como prêmio por bom comportamento	1 2 3
7. Você oferece para a criança um brinquedo ou uma atividade favorita como prêmio por ela comer	1 2 3
8. Você oferece para a criança uma sobremesa especial como prêmio por ela comer	1 2 3
9. Você deixa a criança substituir um alimento por outro que ela goste	1 2 3
10. Você deixa a criança escolher quais alimentos comer, mas apenas entre aqueles que são oferecidos a ela	1 2 3
11. Você prepara uma refeição ou alguma comida especial para a criança, diferente daquela da família	1 2 3
12. Você impede a criança de comer demais	1 2 3
13. Você diz para a criança o quanto você gosta da comida	1 2 3
14. Você diz para a criança que será bom o sabor da comida se ela experimentar	1 2 3
15. Você diz para a criança que seus amigos ou irmãos gostam da comida	1 2 3
16. Você diz para a criança que um alimento vai deixá-lo/la saudável, inteligente e forte	1 2 3
17. Você dá fruta para a criança todos os dias	1 2 3
18. Você faz mudanças na comida da criança para diminuir a quantidade de gordura	1 2 3
19. Você come frutas todos os dias	1 2 3
20. Você come verduras e legumes todos os dias	1 2 3
21. Você toma refrigerante todos os dias	1 2 3
22. Você come balas ou doces todos os dias	1 2 3
23. Você come salgadinho todos os dias	1 2 3
24. Você faz mudanças na sua própria comida para diminuir a quantidade de gordura	1 2 3
25. Você limita o número de doces que a criança pode comer por dia	1 2 3
26. Você limita a quantidade de refrigerante que a criança pode tomar por dia	1 2 3
27. Você limita o número de salgadinhos que a criança pode comer por dia	1 2 3
28. Você diz para a criança comer mesmo se ele/ela diz "não estou com fome"	1 2 3
29. Você insiste para a criança comer quando ele/ela está com sono ou não está se sentindo bem	1 2 3
30. Você insiste para a criança comer quando ele/ela está chateada	1 2 3
31. Você coloca um pouco de cada alimento no prato da criança	1 2 3

TEXTBOX 8.11 SPANISH TRANSLATION OF PMAS

Provided by Stephanie Unger, M.A.
Instructor of Spanish
Penn State University
Schuylkill Campus, PA

Durante una semana típica, ¿con que frecuencia exhibe Ud. cada uno de los siguientes comportamientos?

COMPORTAMIENTO DURANTE LA COMIDA.	1 = NUNCA 2 = A VECES 3 = SIEMPRE		
1. Hace Ud. la comida como un juego para el niño.	1	2	3
2. Come Ud. la misma comida como el niño.	1	2	3
3. Se sienta con el niño pero no come Ud.	1	2	3
4. Permite Ud. al niño comer cualquier comida que quiera.	1	2	3
5. Permite Ud. al niño a poner el sabor a su gusto.	1	2	3
6. Le da al niño la comida favorita por portarse bien.	1	2	3
7. Le ofrece al niño un juguete o actividad favorita por comer bien.	1	2	3
8. Le ofrece un postre especial por comer bien.	1	2	3
9. Le permite sustituir una comida que le gusta más en vez de la comida servida.	1	2	3
10. Le permite al niño escojer una comida pero solamente de las comidas ofrecidas.	1	2	3
11. Le prepara una comida especial diferente de la comida familiar.	1	2	3
12. Deja Ud. el niño de comer demasiado.	1	2	3
13. Le dice cuanto le gusta Ud. la comida.	1	2	3
14. Le dice que la comida tendrá un sabor bueno para probarla.	1	2	3
15. Le dice que sus hermanos les gusta la comida mucho.	1	2	3
16. Le dice que la comida se hace más fuerte, inteligente y sano.	1	2	3
17. Le da fruta al niño cada día.	1	2	3
18. Cambia la dieta del niño para evitar o bajar la grasa.	1	2	3
19. Come Ud. la fruta cada día.	1	2	3
20. Come Ud. vegetales cada día.	1	2	3
21. Bebe Ud. los refrescos todos los días.	1	2	3
22. Come Ud. los dulces todos los días.	1	2	3
23. Come Ud. los antojitos con mucha sal cada día.	1	2	3
24. Ud. cambia su dieta misma para evitar o bajar la grasa.	1	2	3
25. Limite Ud. los dulces que come el niño.	1	2	3
26. Limite Ud. los refrescos que toma el niño cada día.	1	2	3
27. Limite Ud. los antojitos con sal que come el niño cada día.	1	2	3
28. Insiste en que el niño coma aunque el dice "no tengo hambre."	1	2	3
29. Insiste en que él coma cuando tiene sueño o no se siente bien.	1	2	3
30. Insiste Ud. en que él coma cuando él no está de buen humor.	1	2	3
31. Pone un poco de cada comida en el plato del niño.	1	2	3

TEXTBOX 8.12 TURKISH TRANSLATION OF PMAS

Translated by S. Hakan Can, Ph.D.
School of Public Affairs
Penn State University
Schuylkill Campus, PA

Siradan bir hafta boyunca, hangi siklikta yemek zamani eylemi davranisi gostermektesiniz?
Her eylemden sonra uygun numarayi yuvarlak icine aliniz.

Ebeveyn Yemek zamani Eylemleri	1 = hic bir zaman 2 = bazen 3 = herzaman		
1. Yemeyi yemeyi cocuk icin eglenceye yada bir oyuna donusturdum.	1	2	3
2. Cocuga verdigim yemeyi bende yedim	1	2	3
3. Cocukla Masaya oturdum ama ben yemedim	1	2	3
4. Cocugun ne isterse onu yemesine izin verdim	1	2	3
5. Cocugun istedigi sekilde yemeye cesni katmasina izin verdim.	1	2	3
6. Cocuga iyi davranisinin odulu olarak istedigi yiyecegi verdim.	1	2	3
7. Cocuga yemesinin karsiliginda odul olarak sevdigi aktiviteyi yada oyuncak verdim.	1	2	3
8. Cocuga yemesinin karsiliginda sevdigi bir tatliyi odul olarak vermeyi teklif ettim	1	2	3
9. Cocuga sevdigi bir yemekle bu yemegi degistirmesine izin verdim.	1	2	3
10. Cocuga onerdigim yemek seceneklerinden istedigi yemegi secmesine izin verdim.	1	2	3
11. Cocuga, ailemizin yedigi yemeklerden farkli olarak ozel yemek hazirladim.	1	2	3
12. Cocugu cok yemekten alikoydum.	1	2	3
13. Cocuga yemegi ne kadar cok sevdigimi soyledim.	1	2	3
14. Cocuga, eger yemeyi denerse tadinin ne kadar guzel oldugunu farkedecegini soyledim.	1	2	3
15. Cocuga, arkadaslarinin yada kardeslerinin bu yemeyi ne kadar sevdiklerini soyledim.	1	2	3
16. Cocuga yemeyin onu saglikli, akilli ve guclu yapacagini soyledim.	1	2	3
17. Cocuga hergun meyve verdim.	1	2	3
18. Cocugun yemeginde hayvansal yag katkisini azaltici degisiklikler yaptim.	1	2	3
19. Her gun meyve yedim.	1	2	3
20. Her gun sebze yedim.	1	2	3
21. Her gun gazli icecek ictim.	1	2	3
22. Her gun tatli yiyecekler ve seker yedim.	1	2	3
23. Her gun tuzlu atistiricilardan yedim.	1	2	3
24. Kendi yemegimde icindeki hayvansal yaglari azaltici yonde degisiklikler yaptim.	1	2	3
25. Cocugun bir gunde yiyebilecegi tatli yiyeceklere sinir koydum.	1	2	3
26. Cocugun bir gunde icebilecegi gazli iceceklere sinir koydum.	1	2	3
27. Cocugun bir gunde yiyebilecegi tuzlu atistiricilara sinir koydum.	1	2	3
28. Cocuk tokum desede yemek yemesi icin israr ettim.	1	2	3
29. Cocugun uykulu olmasi ve kendini iyi hissememesi durumlarinda ya yemesi icin israr ettim.	1	2	3
30. Cocugun, duygusal olarak uzgun oldugu durumlarda da yemesi icin israr ettim.	1	2	3
31. Her yemekten bir tane cocugun tabagina koydum.	1	2	3

PLATE A–PLATE B HOME INTERVENTION FOR EXTREME PICKY EATERS

While the parent mealtime actions described earlier may be sufficient to encourage most children to develop healthy eating habits, they may not work for children who are extreme picky eaters. These children may also be less likely to benefit from the school-based Kid's Choice Program because they have *never* tasted the healthy FV and drinks included in the program, and because their parents *persist* in sending packed lunches to school that contain only their favorite and familiar foods.

As discussed in earlier chapters, research has documented that children develop preferences for new foods by repeatedly *tasting* those foods (Birch & Marlin, 1982; Birch et al., 1987; Sullivan & Birch, 1990, 1994; Wardle et al., 2003). Looking, touching, and smelling foods is not enough to change food acceptance. However, parents of extreme picky eaters may ask, "How do I get my child to taste a new food enough to develop a preference for new foods when he [or she] refuses even to try them?" In response, our second author has developed the "Plate A–Plate B" technique for parents of extreme picky eaters referred to his Feeding Clinic at Penn State Hershey Medical Center (Pizzo et al., 2012; Seiverling et al., 2012).

The goal of the Plate A–Plate B home intervention for extreme picky eaters is to gradually increase the child's number and size of new food tastes to broaden the child's diet variety so he/she may join in shared meals with the family and during school lunch. The Plate A–Plate B intervention consists of structured meals and snacks during which parents present both new foods on Plate A and familiar favorite foods on Plate B, with the child asked to eat one small bite from Plate A before eating a bite from Plate B. Please see Textbox 8.13 for a summary of parent instructions to deliver the following steps for the Plate A–Plate B intervention:

(1) New food selection:
Prior to starting the intervention, parents must decide which foods they want to introduce to their child. We suggest start-

ing with 20 foods the child does not currently eat, but that are frequently eaten by other family members. These foods should require little effort or chewing from the child, and they may be somewhat similar in taste, color, or texture to foods the child currently accepts.

(2) **Specific time and place for 10-minute meals and snacks:** These meals and snacks are most effective if they are only given in areas used by the family for eating, with three meals and two to three small snacks being sufficient. Parents should set a timer to keep track of the 10 minutes. The child is allowed to have water at any time across the day. Setting up this "eating routine" is important because it eliminates consumption of liquid or snack foods that picky eaters often have between meals, which reduces their motivation to eat foods offered during family meals. The goal of this step is to help the child be hungry when meals and snacks are offered.

(3) **Present Plate A (new foods) and Plate B (familiar foods):** For each 10-minute meal or snack, parents present the child with Plate A, which contains one or two pea-size bites of four new foods. They also present Plate B, which contains three or four foods that are familiar and accepted by the child. A beverage is also available that the child enjoys. Parents tell the child, "Take a bite from Plate A [pointing to it], then you may have a bite from Plate B [pointing to it] and have a drink." Parents should calmly wait for the child to accept a bite from Plate A while ignoring crying or refusal, repeating the rule approximately every 30 seconds. If the child eats a bite from Plate A and then spits out the food, parents do not give a bite from Plate B or a drink, but they offer another bite from Plate A. When the timer rings, the child may leave the table. If the timer rings and the child is still eating, he/she may continue to eat while following the Plate A–Plate B rules.

(4) **Offer praise or other small incentives for trying new foods:**
As soon as the child eats a bite from Plate A, parents praise the child and offer both the drink and a bite from Plate B. For most children this is sufficient. For some children, other incentives

may be offered such as token rewards (stars on a chart, buttons in a jar) that can be accumulated and traded in for items and activities the child enjoys. These incentives may be earned for accepting bites of food from Plate A, but incentives have also been used to improve sitting in the chair quietly, not throwing food, and other appropriate mealtime behaviors. Incentives may also be immediately available such as the parent reading or spending other one-on-one time with the child after the meal, or the child earning additional television, video game, or computer time. Incentives should be no cost or low cost. Initially the incentives should be easy for the child to earn.

(5) **Ignore inappropriate behaviors (crying, complaining, gagging):**

It is very important that parents avoid rewarding inappropriate behaviors with attention and escape from the Plate A–Plate B intervention. Parents can simply repeat, "Take one bite from Plate A, then you may have one bite from Plate B and have a drink." If the child leaves the table, parents simply end that meal's intervention, then repeat the process at the next meal or snack. Parents will need to be patient because our research has shown that as children taste more and more new foods, the process becomes easier, often to the point that children are requesting new foods.

(6) **Increase bite sizes across meals:**

Initially, the bites offered on Plate A will be the size of a pea. When the child is eating pea-size bites of a particular food without complaining for three consecutive meals, parents can increase them to half spoonful–size bites. When the child is eating the half spoonful–size bites easily for three consecutive meals, parents can increase them to spoonful-sized bites. The child's progress of new food acceptance can be recorded with the Datasheet to Record New Food Acceptance at Home (see Textbox 8.14). It can be used to keep track of each new food offered to the child on Plate A, the size of bites accepted, the number of consecutive meals the child has accepted each food, and the point for each food when the child no longer needs presentation of the back-up Plate B of previous favorite foods.

(7) Use these between-meal procedures:

While parents are presenting the Plate A–Plate B intervention to their picky eater, the child is allowed as much water as he/she desires between meals. The child may also have any of the new foods from Plate A, but none of his/her original favorite foods. If the child ate nothing or only a small amount at a particular meal, that is fine because it increases the child's hunger motivation to try new foods at the next meal or snack. Some meals will be more difficult than others, especially in the beginning.

(8) Fade the Plate A–Plate B intervention:

Ultimately, the goal of the intervention is that the child eat foods from family meals without the need for any special treatment. As new foods are repeatedly offered and tasted during the Plate A–Plate B meals, the child will begin to eat some foods without resistance, often eating several bites in a row without needing to follow them with bites from Plate B, and even asking for these foods outside of meals. Once the child is eating spoonful-size bites of several new foods without difficulty, parents may begin to offer two or three of them at meal or snack times without the need of Plate B. Over time, more and more of the child's meals and snacks will consist of just a single plate, rather than Plate A and Plate B.

TEXTBOX 8.13 PARENT INSTRUCTIONS FOR PLATE A–PLATE B INTERVENTION

STEP 1: Select new foods

Select approximately 20 foods that your child does not currently eat but that are frequently eaten and enjoyed by other family members. It may help to choose foods that are somewhat similar in taste, color, or texture to those the child currently eats.

STEP 2: Set specific times for 10-minute meals and snacks

Select times and places for approximately three meals and two to three snacks, setting a timer for 10 minutes. You are trying to make eating and trying new foods a *habit* for your child.

STEP 3: Present Plate A (new foods) and Plate B (familiar foods)

For each meal or snack, present Plate A with one or two pea-size bites of four new foods and Plate B with three or four foods that are currently eaten by the child. A beverage the child enjoys should also be made available. Tell the child, "Take a bite from Plate A [pointing to it], then you may have a bite from Plate B [pointing to it] and have a drink." Repeat the rule about every 30 seconds until your child takes a bite. When the timer rings, your child may leave the table or continue to eat if following the Plate A–Plate B rules.

STEP 4: Offer praise or small incentives for trying new foods

When the child eats a bite from Plate A, praise the child and offer a bite from Plate B and a drink. For most children, just the alternation between the new food and the familiar food is enough to increase willingness to try the new foods. However, additional incentives can be offered using a token reward system (stars on a chart, buttons in a jar, points on a calendar) that can be accumulated and traded for items and activities the child enjoys. While tokens have been used to reward tasting new foods, tokens have also been used to reward coming to the table without complaining, sitting quietly at table, and other appropriate eating behaviors.

STEP 5: **Ignore inappropriate behaviors (crying, gagging)**

Remain calm and ignore inappropriate behaviors such as crying, complaining, or food refusal. Many children have learned to exhibit inappropriate behavior to avoid eating new foods, so these behaviors will gradually go away if ignored. Simply repeat to your child, "Take one bite from Plate A, then you may have one bite from Plate B and have a drink." If the child leaves the table, end the meal and repeat the process at the next meal or snack. As children taste more and more new foods, the process of tasting becomes easier, often to the point that children begin requesting new foods.

STEP 6: **Increase bite sizes across meals**

Initially, the bites offered on Plate A will be the size of a pea. When the child is eating pea-size bites of a food without difficulty for three consecutive meals, increase the size to half spoonful–size bites, then to spoonful-size bites. The child's progress can be recorded with the Datasheet to Record New Food Acceptance at Home (see Textbox 8.14).

STEP 7: **Use these between-meal procedures**

Between meals, allow the child to have as much water as he/she desires and any of the new foods from Plate A, but none of the original favorite foods.

STEP 8: **Fade the Plate A–Plate B intervention**

As new foods are repeatedly offered and tasted, the child will begin to eat some foods without resistance, often eating several bites without following them with bites from Plate B, and even asking for them outside of meals. Once your child is eating spoonful-size bites of several new foods without difficulty, you may begin to offer two or three of them at meal or snack times without the need of Plate B.

TEXTBOX 8.14 DATASHEET TO RECORD NEW FOOD ACCEPTANCE AT HOME

For each Plate A (new food)–Plate B (familiar food) meal, mark the box to show child's acceptance of each new food: 0 = no bite, 1 = pea-size bite, 2 = half-spoon bite, 3 = spoon-size bite

Meals

New Food	1	2	3	4	5	6	7	8	9	10

9

WHEN TO SEEK PROFESSIONAL HELP

Although the school-based Kids' Choice Program (Chapter 4) and recommended parent mealtime actions (Chapter 8) can help most children develop healthier eating patterns, some children may still need assistance from healthcare providers. The purpose of this section is to provide guidelines for school personnel and parents about how to identify children's feeding problems and when to seek assistance from pediatricians or other healthcare providers including special feeding programs.

MEASURING CHILDREN'S FEEDING PROBLEMS

Research suggests that at least 25% of children will experience some type of feeding problem during childhood (Manikam & Perman, 2000). Children with special needs such as autism or other developmental disabilities have a higher risk for feeding problems (Lukens & Linscheid, 2008; Schreck et al., 2004), but approximately 30% of children referred to hospital feeding clinics have no special needs other than their feeding problems (Field et al., 2003; Williams, Hendy, and Knecht, 2008). Despite such widespread occurrence of feeding problems in children, little attention has been paid to measurement of the dimensions or subtypes of such child feeding problems.

Available measures of child feeding problems include the Child Eating Behavior Questionnaire (Wardle et al., 2001) and the Behavioral Pediatric Feeding Assessment Scale (Crist & Napier-Phillips, 2001). Although these measures cover a range of feeding problems (such as poor appetite, limited food variety, slowness in eating, excessive drinking), none of them includes measurement of disruptive behaviors such as aggressive behavior or self-injurious behavior, which often accompany children's picky eating and prompt parents to give up and serve children only "special meals" of their favorite foods (Kerwin, 1999; Linscheid, 2006; Rhoe et al., 2006).

One recent measure of child feeding problems that was developed to include disruptive behaviors is the Brief Assessment of Mealtime Behaviors in Children (BAMBIC) (Hendy et al., 2013). The 10-item BAMBIC was developed with a sample of 202 feeding-clinic children that included 60 children with autism spectrum disorders, 85 children with other special needs, and 57 children of average development. The BAMBIC identified three dimensions of child feeding problems: food refusal, limited variety, and disruptive behavior. Although the two special-needs groups of children showed higher mean scores for food refusal than did average-developing children in the feeding clinic, all three diagnostic groups showed similar mean scores for limited variety and disruptive behavior.

Please see Textbox 9.1 for the BAMBIC, Textbox 9.2 for BAMBIC scoring instructions, and Textbox 9.3 for BAMBIC norms for feeding-clinic children in the three diagnostic groups (autism, other special needs, average developing). Although BAMBIC norms are not yet available for average-developing children who have *not* been referred to a feeding clinic, the norms for average-developing children in the feeding clinic may be used as a "level of concern" for parents, who may then wish to seek professional help for their children's feeding problems.

WHEN AND WHERE TO SEEK PROFESSIONAL HELP

Children's feeding problems can range in severity from minor conditions that do not impact the child's health or family functioning, to severe conditions that can adversely affect the child's health and development and disrupt mealtimes and other areas of family functioning. In many cases, parents realize their child is having a problem with eating, but they are unsure about what they can do or which professionals can help their child.

One obvious indicator of children's feeding problems is lack of growth or insufficient growth, information that most schools gather at least annually for all students. Some schools report children's body mass index percentile scores (BMI%) to parents of all of their students, while other schools report this information only for children with BMI% scores under the 10th percentile or greater than the 85th percentile. Because both underweight and overweight children have increased risks for a variety of health problems (Blössner & Onis, 2005; CDC, 2000; Must & Strauss, 1999), the school nurse typically sends recommendations to parents that they should discuss their children's growth with their primary care provider.

Many children who eat an extremely limited variety of foods (see BAMBIC dimension "limited variety") have increased risks for health problems and yet can still be in the normal weight range (with BMI% scores between the 10th and 85th percentile). A common nutritional deficit in picky eaters is iron-deficient anemia, which can result from eating too few iron-rich foods (such as red meats, green leafy vegetables, iron-fortified cereals or breads) and from eating too many dairy products because the calcium in dairy products blocks iron absorption. Picky eaters may also be deficient in vitamins A and C, which can result in corneal erosions, scurvy, and limb pain (Williams & Seiverling, 2010).

In addition to health risks, picky eating habits may also have an adverse effect on family functioning such as disrupting meals with power struggles over food (see BAMBIC dimensions of "food refusal" and "disruptive behavior") or making the family feel too embarrassed by the child's behavior to eat in public settings. For example, one study compared the mealtime interactions of parents and children with and without feeding problems, finding that children with feeding problems showed significantly more complaining and non-compliant behaviors, and their parents showed more negative and coercive behaviors (Sanders et al., 1993).

While your local hospital may be able to provide clinical resources for the treatment of children's overweight and feeding problems, specialized services for children with feeding problems may be more difficult to locate. Please see Textbox 9.4 for names and contact information for a number of feeding programs throughout the United States that may serve as resources, or go to the website www.oley.org/feeding_programs.

TEXTBOX 9.1 BRIEF ASSESSMENT OF MEALTIME BEHAVIOR IN CHILDREN (BAMBIC)

Think about mealtimes with your child during the past 6 months. Please circle the appropriate number to rate how often the behavior occurs.

CHILD MEALTIME BEHAVIOR	1 = never, almost never 2 = seldom 3 = occasionally 4 = often 5 = almost every meal
1. My child cries or screams during mealtimes.	1 2 3 4 5
2. My child turns his/her face or body away from food.	1 2 3 4 5
3. My child is aggressive during mealtimes (hitting, kicking, scratching).	1 2 3 4 5
4. My child shows self-injurious behavior at meals (scratching, biting self).	1 2 3 4 5
5. My child is disruptive during mealtimes (pushing, throwing things).	1 2 3 4 5
6. My child closes his/her mouth tightly when food is presented.	1 2 3 4 5
7. My child is willing to try new foods.	1 2 3 4 5
8. My child dislikes certain foods and will not eat them.	1 2 3 4 5
9. My child prefers the same foods at each meal.	1 2 3 4 5
10. My child accepts or prefers a variety of foods.	1 2 3 4 5

TEXTBOX 9.2 SCORING THREE BAMBIC DIMENSIONS

Steps:
(1) For each BAMBIC dimension, record ratings for all items in the dimension.
(2) Sum all ratings in the dimension (using *reversed* scores as indicated below).
(3) Divide the sum by the number of items in the dimension.

FOOD REFUSAL:
Ratings: _____ + _____ + _____ = _____ (Sum)
Item #:   1   2   6
Food refusal score is this sum divided by 3 = _____

LIMITED VARIETY:
First, reverse ratings for items 7 and 10 (only) so that 1 = 5, 2 = 4, 3 = 3, 4 = 2, 5 = 1.
(new) Ratings: _____ + _____ + _____ + _____ = _____ (Sum)
Item #:   7   8   9   10
Limited variety score is this sum divided by 4 = _____

DISRUPTIVE BEHAVIOR:
Ratings: _____ + _____ + _____ = _____ (Sum)
Item #:   3   4   5
Disruptive behavior score is this sum divided by 3 = ___

TEXTBOX 9.3 NORMS FOR THREE BAMBIC DIMENSIONS

Note: Values shown are mean 5-point ratings for child behavior (1 = never or almost never, 2 = seldom, 3 = occasionally, 4 = often, 5 = almost every meal) as reported by parents of children referred to a hospital-based feeding clinic.

BAMBIC DIMENSION	Average-developing children ($n = 57$) MEAN (SD)	Children with autism ($n = 60$) MEAN (SD)	Children with other special needs ($n = 85$) MEAN (SD)
Food Refusal	2.67 (1.01)	2.97 (1.01)	3.07 (1.04)
Limited Variety	4.04 (1.01)	4.30 (1.03)	3.94 (0.99)
Disruptive Behavior	1.63 (0.88)	2.03 (1.12)	1.73 (0.86)

TEXTBOX 9.4 CLINICS TREATING CHILDREN WITH FEEDING PROBLEMS

ORGANIZATION	LOCATION	WEBSITE
Clinic 4 Kidz	Sausalito, CA	www.clinic4kidz.com
The Children's Hospital	Denver, CO	www.thechildrenshospital.org
Marcus Institute	Atlanta, GA	www.marcus.org
University of Iowa Children's Hospital	Iowa City, IA	www.uihealthcare.com
St. Mary's Feeding Disorders Program	Evansville, IN	www.stmarys.org
University of Kansas Feeding Clinic	Kansas City, KS	www.kumc.edu/cchd/clinic_feeding
Kennedy Krieger Institute	Baltimore, MD	www.feedingdisorders.kennedykrieger.org
Helen DeVos Children's Hospital	Grand Rapids, MI	www.helendevoschildrens.org
Munroe-Meyer Institute	Omaha, NE	www.unmc.edu/mmi
St. Joseph's Children's Hospital	Patterson, NJ	www.feedingcenter.org
St. Mary's Hospital for Children	Bayside, NY	www.stmaryskids.org
Children's Institute of Pittsburgh	Pittsburgh, PA	www.amazingkids.org
Penn State Hershey Feeding Program	Hershey, PA	www.pennstatehershey.org
Texas Children's Hospital	Houston, TX	www.texaschildrens.org
Kluge Children's Rehabilitation Center	Charlottesville, VA	www.healthsystem.virginia.edu
Seattle Children's Hospital	Seattle, WA	www.seattlechildrens.org

Note: This list is not comprehensive and is not an endorsement of any particular program listed. A more comprehensive listing can be found at www.oley.org/feeding_programs.

REFERENCES

American Dietetic Association. (ADA). (2000). Local support for nutrition integrity in schools. *Journal of the American Dietetic Association, 100,* 108–111.

Andersen, R. E., Crespo, C. J., Bartlett, S. J., Cheskin, L. J., & Pratt, M. (1998). Relationship of physical activity and television watching with body weight and level of fatness among children: Results from the Third National Health and Nutrition Examination Survey. *Journal of the American Medical Association, 279,* 938–942.

Bandura, A. (1997). *Self-efficacy: The exercise of control.* New York: Freeman & Company.

Baranowski, T., Davis, M., Resnicow, K., Baranowski, J., Doyle, C., Lin, L. S., Smith, M., & Wang, D. T. (2000). Gimme 5 fruit, juice and vegetables for fun and health: Outcome evaluation. *Health Education and Behavior, 27,* 96–111.

Batsell, W. R., Brown, A. S., Ansfield, M. E., & Paschall, G. Y. (2002). "You will eat all of that!": A retrospective analysis of forced consumption episodes. *Appetite, 38,* 211–219.

Bauer, K. W., Yang, Y. W., & Austin, S. B. (2004). "How can we stay healthy when you're throwing all of this in front of us?" Findings from focus groups and interviews in middle schools on environmental influences on nutrition and physical activity. *Health Education and Behavior, 31,* 34–36.

Baughcum, A. E., Powers, S. W., Johnson, S. B., Chamberlin, L. A., Deeks, C. M., Jain, A., & Whitaker, R. C. (2001). Maternal feeding practices and beliefs and their relationships to overweight in early childhood. *Journal of Developmental and Behavioral Pediatrics, 22,* 391–408.

Baxter, S. D., & Thompson, W. O. (2002). Fourth-grade children's consumption of fruit and vegetable items available as part of school lunches is closely related to preferences. *Journal of Nutrition Education and Behavior, 34,* 166–171.

Bellisle, F., Rolland–Cachera, M. F., & Kellogg Scientific Advisory Committee on Child and Nutrition (2000). Three consecutive (1993, 1995, 1997) surveys of food intake, nutritional attitudes and knowledge, and lifestyle in 1,000 French children, aged 9–11 years. *Journal of Human Nutrition and Dietetics, 13,* 101–111.

Birch, L. L. (1979). Preschool children's food preferences and consumption patterns. *Journal of Nutrition Education, 11,* 189–192.

Birch, L. L., Birch, D., Marlin, D., & Kramer, L. (1982). Effects of instrumental consumption on children's food preference. *Appetite, 3,* 125–134.

Birch, L. L., Fisher, J. O., Grimm-Thomas, K., Markey, C. N., Sawyer, R., & Johnson, S. L. (2001). Confirmatory factor analysis of the child feeding questionnaire: A measure of parental attitudes, beliefs and practices about child feeding and obesity proneness. *Appetite, 36,* 201–210.

Birch, L. L., & Marlin, D. W. (1982). I don't like it; never tried it: Effects of exposure on two-year-old children's food preferences. *Appetite, 3,* 353–360.

Birch, L. L., Marlin, D. W., & Rotter, J. (1984). Eating as the "means" activity in a contingency: Effects on young children's food preferences. *Child Development, 55,* 532–539.

Birch, L. L., McPhee, L., Shoba, B. C., Pirok, E., & Stineberg, L. (1987). What kind of exposure reduces children's food neophobia: Looking vs. tasting? *Appetite, 9,* 171–178.

Blanchette, L., & Brug, J. (2005). Determinants of fruit and vegetable consumption among 6–12-year-old children and effective interventions to increase consumption. *Journal of Human Nutrition and Diet, 18,* 431–443.

Blössner, M., & Onis, M. (2005). *Malnutrition: Environmental Burden of Disease Series.* Geneva: World Health Organization.

Brown, J. E., Nicholson, J. M., Broom, D. H., & Bittman, M. (2011). Television viewing by school-aged children: Associations with physical activity, snack food consumption, and unhealthy weight. *Social Indicators Research, 101,* 221–225.

Bryant–Waugh, R., Markham, L., Kreipe, R., & Walsh, B. T. (in press). Feeding and eating disorders in childhood. *International Journal of Eating Disorders.*

Budd, G. M., & Volpe, S. L. (2006). School-based obesity prevention: Research, challenges, and recommendations. *Journal of School Health, 76,* 485–496.

Burchett, H. (2003). Increasing fruit and vegetable consumption among British primary school children: A review. *Health Education, 103,* 99–109.

Carruth, B. R., Skinner, J., Houck, K., Moran, J., Coletta, F., & Ott, D. (1998). The phenomenon of "picky eater": A behavioral marker in eating patterns of toddlers. *Journal of American College of Nutrition, 17,* 180–186.

Carruth, B. R., Ziegler, P. J., Gordon, A., & Barr, S. I. (2004). Prevalence of "picky/fussy" eaters among infants and toddlers and their caregivers' decision about offering new food. *Journal of the American Dietetic Association, 104,* S57–S64.

Centers for Disease Control and Prevention. CDC. (2000). *School health index for physical activity and health eating: A self-assessment and planning guide.* Atlanta, GA: author.

Cole, T. J., Bellizzi, M. C., Flegal, K. M., & Dietz, W. H. (2000). Establishing a standard definition for child overweight and obesity world-wide: International survey. *British Medical Journal, 320,* 1–6.

Contento, I. R., Balch, G. I., & Bronner, Y. L. (1995). The effectiveness of nutrition education and implications for nutrition education, policy, programs, and research: A review of research. *Journal of Nutrition Education, 27,* 277–418.

Cooke, L. J. (2007). The importance of exposure for healthy eating in childhood: A review. *Journal of Human Nutrition and Dietetics, 20,* 294–301.

Cooke, L. J., Chambers, L. C., Afiez, E. V., Croker, H. A., Boniface, D., Yeomans, M. R., & Wardle, J. (2011). Eating for pleasure or profit: The effect of incentives on children's enjoyment of vegetables. *Psychological Science, 22,* 190–196.

Cooke, L., & Wardle, J. (2005). Age and gender differences in children's food preferences. *British Journal of Nutrition, 93,* 741–746.

Cooke, L., Wardle, J., Gibson, E. L., Sapochik, M., Sheiham, A., & Lawson, M. (2004). Demographic, familial, and trait predictors of fruit and vegetable consumption by preschool children. *Public Health and Nutrition, 7,* 295–302.

Costanzo, P. R., & Woody, E. (1985). Domain-specific parenting styles and their impact on the child's development of particular deviance: The example of obesity proneness. *Journal of Social and Clinical Psychology, 3,* 425–445.

Crist, W., & Napier-Phillips, A. (2001). Mealtime behaviors of young children: A comparison of normative and clinical data. *Journal of Developmental and Behavioral Pediatrics, 22,* 279–286.

Cullen, K. W., Baranowski, T., Owens, E., Marsh, T., Rittenberry, L, & de Moor, C. (2003). Availability, accessibility, and preferences for fruit, 100% fruit juice, and vegetables influence children's dietary behavior. *Health, Education, and Behavior, 30,* 615–626.

Cullen, K. W., Eagan, J., & Baranowski, T. (2000). Effect of a al carte and snack bar foods at school on children's lunchtime intake of fruits and vegetables. *Journal of the American Dietetic Association, 100,* 1482–1486.

Darmon, N., & Drewnowski, A. (2008). Does social class predict diet quality? *American Journal of Clinical Nutrition, 87,* 1107–1117.

Davis, M., Baranowski, T., Resnicow, K., Baranowski, J., Doyle, C., Smith, M., Wang, D. T., Yaroch, A., & Hebert, D. (2000). Gimme 5 fruit and vegetables for fun and health: Process evaluation. *Health Education and Behavior, 27,* 167–176.

Davison, K. K., & Birch, L. L. (2001). Weight status, parent reaction, and self-concept in five-year-old girls. *Pediatrics, 107,* 46–53.

Deci, E. L., & Ryan, R. M. (1985). *Intrinsic motivation and self-determination in human behavior.* New York: Plenum.

Deckelbaum, R. J., & Williams, C. L. (2001). Childhood obesity: The health issue. *Obesity Research, 9*(Suppl. 4), 239S–243S.

Diehl, J. M. (1999). Food preferences of 10- to 14-year-old boys and girls. *Schweizerische Medizinische Wochenschrift, 129,* 151–161.

DiMeglio, D. P., & Mattes, R. D. (2000). Liquid versus solid carbohydrate: Effects on food intake and body weight. *International Journal of Obesity and Related Metabolic Disorders, 24,* 794–800.

Dovey, T. M., Staples, P. A., Gibson, E. L., & Halford, J. C. G. (2008). Food neophobia and "picky/fussy" eating in children: A review. *Appetite, 50,* 181–193.

Drewnawski, A. (1997). Taste preferences and food intake. *Annual Review of Nutrition, 17,* 237–253.

Duncker, K. (1938). Experimental modification of children's food preferences through social suggestion. *The Journal of Abnormal and Social Psychology, 33,* 489–507.

Edwards, J. S. A., & Hartwell, H. H. (2002). Fruit and vegetable attitudes and knowledge of primary school children. *Journal of Human Nutrition and Dietetics, 15,* 365–374.

Eisenberger, R., & Cameron, J. (1996). Detrimental effects of reward. *American Psychologist, 51,* 1153–1166.

Faith, M. S., Scanlon, K. S., Birch, L. L., Francis, L. A., & Sherry, B. (2004). Parent-child feeding strategies and their relationships to child eating and weight status. *Obesity Research, 12,* 1711–1722.

Falciglia, G. A., Couch, S. C., Gribble, L. S., Pabst, S. M., & Frank, R. (2000). Food neophobia in childhood affects diet variety. *Journal of American Dietary Association, 100,* 1474–1481.

Field, D., Garland, M., & Williams, K. (2003). Correlates of specific childhood feeding problems. *Journal of Pediatrics and Child Health, 39,* 299–304.

Fisher, J. O., & Birch, L. L. (1999). Restricting access to foods and children's eating. *Appetite, 32,* 405–419.

Flood-Obbagy, J. E., & Rolls, B. J. (2009). The effect of fruit in different forms on energy intake and satiety at a meal. *Appetite, 52,* 416–422.

Galloway, A. T., Fiorito, L. M., Lee, Y., & Birch, L. L. (2005). Parental pressure, dietary patterns and weight status among girls who are "picky/fussy" eaters. *Journal of the American Dietetic Association, 103,* 692–698.

Gleason, P., & Suitor, C. (2000). *Changes in children's diets: 1989–91 to 1994–96.* Washington, DC: United States Department of Agriculture.

Grimmett, C., Croker, H., Carnell, S., & Wardle, J. (2008). Telling parents their child's weight status: Psychological impact of a weight-screening program. *Pediatrics, 122,* 682–688.

Harper, L. V., & Sanders, K. M. (1975). The effects of adults' eating on young children's acceptance of unfamiliar foods. *Journal of Experimental Child Psychology, 20,* 206–214.

Harris, J. L., Bargh, J. A., & Brownell, K. D. (2009). Priming effects of television food advertising on eating behavior. *Health Psychology, 28,* 404–413.

Harris, J. R. (1995). Where is the child's environment? A group socialization theory of development. *Psychological Review, 102,* 458–489.

Hendy, H. M. (1999). Comparison of five teacher actions to encourage children's new food acceptance. *Annals of Behavioral Medicine, 21,* 20–26.

———. (2002). Effectiveness of trained peer models to encourage food acceptance in preschool children. *Appetite, 39,* 217–225.

Hendy, H. M., & Raudenbush, B. (2000). Effectiveness of teacher modeling to encourage food acceptance in preschool children. *Appetite, 33,* 61–76.

Hendy, H. M., & Williams, K. E. (2012). Mother's feeding practices for children 3 to 10 years of age and their associations with child demographics. *Appetite, 58,* 710–716.

Hendy, H. M., Williams, K. E., & Camise, T. S. (2005). "Kid's Choice" school lunch program increases children's fruit and vegetable acceptance. *Appetite, 45,* 250–263.

———. (2011). Kid's Choice Program improves weight management behaviors and weight status in school children. *Appetite, 56,* 484–494.

———. (2012). Kid's Choice Program increases healthy food choices by fussy-eating children during school lunch. In L. V. Bernardt (Ed.), *Advances in Medicine and Biology, Volume 28* (pp. 299–308). Hauppauge, NY: Nova Science Publishers.

Hendy, H. M., Williams, K. E., Camise, T. S., Alderman, S., Ivy, J., & Reed, J. (2007). Overweight and average-weight children equally responsive to "Kid's Choice Program" to increase fruit and vegetable consumption. *Appetite, 49,* 683–686.

Hendy, H. M., Williams, K. E., Camise, T. S., Eckman, N., & Hedemann, A. (2009). The Parent Mealtime Action Scale (PMAS): Development and association with children's diet and weight. *Appetite, 52,* 328–339.

Hendy, H. M., Williams, K. E., Camise, T. S., Rahn, D., Costigan, C., Gaskins, S., & Moyer, C. (2009). Kid's Choice Program improves two weight management behaviors in school children. In F. Columbus (Ed.), *Vegetables and Health.* Hauppauge, NY: Nova Science Publishers.

Hendy, H. M., Seiverling, L., Lukens, C. T., and Williams, K. E., (2013). The Brief Assessment of Mealtime Behaviors in Children: Psychometrics and association with child characteristics and parent responses. *Children's Health Care, 42,* 1–14.

Hendy, H. M., Williams, K. E., Riegel, K., & Paul, C. (2010). Parent mealtime actions that mediate associations between children's fussy eating and their weight and diet. *Appetite, 54,* 191–195.

Hernandez, B., Gortmaker, S. L., Colditz, G. A., Peterson, K. E., Laird, N. M., & Para-Cabrera, S. (1999). Association of obesity with physical activity, television programs and other forms of video viewing among children in Mexico City. *International Journal of Obesity, 23,* 845–854.

Hitt, D. D., Marriott, R. G., & Esser, J. K. (1992). Effects of delayed rewards and task interest on intrinsic motivation. *Basic and Applied Social Psychology, 13,* 405–414.

Horne, P. J., Fergus-Lowe, C. F., Fleming, P. F. J., & Dowey, A. J. (1995). An effective procedure for changing food preferences in five to seven year old children. *Proceedings of the Nutrition Society, 54,* 441–452.

Horne, P. J., Greenhalgh, J., Erjavec, M., Lowe, C. F., Viktor, S., & Whitaker, C. J. (2011). Increasing pre-school children's consumption of fruit and vegetables. A modeling and rewards intervention. *Appetite, 56,* 375–385.

Howerton, M. W., Bell, B. S., Dodd, K. W., Berrigan, D., Stozenberg-Solomon, R., & Nebeling, L. (2007). School-based nutrition programs produced a moderate increase in fruit and vegetable consumption: Meta and pooling analyses from seven studies. *Journal of Nutrition Education and Behavior, 39,* 186–196.

Hughes, S. O., Shewchuck, R. M., Baskin, M. L., Nicklas, T. A., & Qu, H. (2008). Indulgent feeding style and children's weight status in preschool. *Journal of Development and Behavioral Pediatrics, 29,* 403–410.

Jahns, L., Siega-Riz, A. M., & Popkin, B. M. (2001). The increasing prevalence of snacking among US children from 1977 to 1996. *Journal of Pediatrics, 138,* 493–498.

James, D., Rienzo, B., & Franzee, C. (1996). Using focus group interviews to understand school meal choices. *Journal of School Health, 66,* 128–131.

Jones, L. R., Steer, C. D., Rogers, I. S., & Emmett, P. M. (2010). Influences on child fruit and vegetable intake: Sociodemographic, parental, and child factors in a longitudinal cohort study. *Public Health Nutrition, 13,* 1122–1130.

Kerwin, M. L. (1999). Empirically supported treatments in pediatric psychology: Severe feeding problems. *Journal of Pediatric Psychology, 24,* 193–214.

Knai, C., Pomerlau, J., Lock, K., & McKee, M. (2006). Getting children to eat more fruit and vegetables: A systematic review. *Preventive Medicine, 42,* 85–95.

Kohn, A. (1993). *Punished by rewards: The trouble with gold stars, incentive plans, A's, praise, and other bribes.* Boston: Houghton Mifflin.

Kroller, K., & Warschburger, P. (2008). Associations between maternal feeding style and food intake of children with a higher risk for overweight. *Appetite, 51,* 166–172.

Latner, J. D., & Stunkard, A. J. (2003). Getting worse: The stigmatization of obese children. *Obesity Research, 11,* 452–456.

Lepper, M. R., Green, D., & Nisbett, R. E. (1973). Undermining children's intrinsic interest with extrinsic reward: A test of the "overjustification" hypothesis. *Journal of Personality and Social Psychology, 28,* 129–137.

Linscheid, T. R. (2006). Behavioral treatments for pediatric feeding disorders. *Behavior Modification, 30,* 6–23.

Lobstein, T., & Dibb, S. (2005). Evidence of a possible link between obesogenic food advertising and child overweight. *Obesity Reviews, 6,* 203–208.

Lockner, D. W., Crowe, T. K., & Skipper, B. J. (2008). Dietary intake and parent's perception of mealtime behaviors in preschool-age children with autism spectrum disorder and in typically developing children. *Journal of the American Dietetic Association, 108,* 1360–1363.

Ludwig, D., Peterson, K. E., & Gortmaker, S. L. (2001). Relation between consumption of sugar-sweetened drinks and childhood obesity: A prospective, observational analysis. *The Lancet, 357,* 505–508.

Lukens, C. T., & Linscheid, T. R. (2008). Development and validation of an inventory to assess mealtime behavior problems in children with autism. *Journal of Autism and Developmental Disorders, 38,* 342–352.

Lytle, L. A., Siefert, S., Greenstein, J., and McGovern, P. (2000). How do children's eating patterns and food choices change over time: Results from a chart study. *American Journal of Health Promotion.* 14, 222–228.

Maier, A., Chabanet, C., Schaal, B., Issanchou, S., & Leathwood, P. (2007). Effects of repeated exposure on acceptance of initially disliked vegetables in 7-month old infants. *Food Quality and Preference, 18,* 1023–1032.

Manikam, S., & Perman, J. (2000). Pediatric feeding disorders. *Journal of Clinical Gastroenterology, 30,* 34–46.

Marchi, M., & Cohen, P. (1990). Early childhood eating behaviors and adolescent eating disorders. *Journal of the American Academy of Child and Adolescent Psychiatry, 29,* 112–117.

Marinho, H. (1942). Social influence in the formation of enduring preferences. *Journal of Abnormal and Social Psychology, 37,* 448–468.

Marples, C. A., & Spillman, D. (1995). Factors affecting students' participation in the Cincinnati public school lunch program. *Adolescence, 30,* 745–754.

Maynard, L. M., Galuska, D. A., Glanck, H. M., & Serdula, M. K. (2003). Maternal perceptions of weight status of children. *Pediatrics, 111*(Part 2), 1226–1231.

McDermott, B., Mamun, A. A., Najman, J. M., Williams, G. M., Callaghan, M. J., & Bor, W. (2010). Longitudinal correlates of the persistence of irregular eating from age 5 to 14 years. *Acta Paediatrica, 99,* 68–71.

McIntosh, W. A., & Zey, M. (1989). Women as gatekeepers of food consumption: A sociological critique. *Food and Foodways, 34,* 317–332.

Mendoza, J. A., Zimmerman, F. J., & Christakis, D. A. (2007). Television viewing, computer use, obesity, and adiposity in US preschool children. *International Journal of Behavioral Nutrition and Physical Activity, 4,* 44. doi: 10.1186/1479–5868-4-44

Mennella, J., Jagnow, C. P., & Beauchamp, G. K. (2001). Prenatal and postnatal flavor learning by human infants. *Pediatrics, 107,* e88.

Mikkila, V., Rasanen, L., Raitakari, O. T., Pietinen, P., & Viikari, J. (2004). Longitudinal changes in diet from childhood into adulthood with respect to risk of cardiovascular diseases: The Caridovascular Risk in Young Finns Study. *European Journal of Clinical Nutrition, 58,* 1038–1045.

Mo-suwan, L., Pongprapai, S., Junjana, C., & Puetpaiboon, A. (1998). Effects of a controlled trial of a school-based exercise program on the obesity indexes of preschool children. *American Journal of Clinical Nutrition, 68,* 1006–1011.

Must, A., & Strauss, R. S. (1999). Risks and consequences of childhood and adolescent obesity. *International Journal of Obesity and Related Metabolic Disorders, 23*(Suppl. 2), S2–S11.

Newman, J., & Layton, B. D. (1984). Overjustification: A self-perception perspective. *Personality and Social Psychology Bulletin, 10,* 419–425.

Newman, J., & Taylor, A. (1992). Effect of a means-end contingency on young children's food preferences. *Journal of Experimental Child Psychology, 55,* 431–439.

Pangrazi, R. P., Beighle, A., Vehige, T., & Vack, C. (2003). Impact of Promoting Lifestyle Activity in Youth (PLAY) on children's activity. *Journal of School Health, 73,* 317–321.

Paul, C., Williams, K. E., Riegel, K., & Gibbons, B. (2007). Combining repeated taste exposure and escape prevention: An intervention for the treatment of extreme food selectivity. *Appetite, 49,* 708–711.

Perez-Rodrigo, C., Rivas, L., Serra-Majem, L., & Aranceta, J. (2003). Food preferences of Spanish children and young people: The enKid study. *European Journal of Clinical Nutrition, 57* (Suppl. 1), S45–48.

Perry, C. L., Bishop, D. B., Taylor, G. L., Davis, M., Story, M., Gray, C., Bishop, S. C., Mays, R. A. W., Lytle, L. A., & Harnack, L. (2004). A randomized school trial of environmental strategies to encourage fruit and vegetable consumption among children. *Health Education and Behavior, 31,* 65–76.

Perry, C. L., Bishop, D. B., Taylor, G., Murray, D. M., Mays, R. W., Dudovitz, B. S., Smyth, M., & Story, M. (1998). Changing fruit and vegetable consumption among children: The 5-a-Day Power Plus program in St. Paul, Minnesota. *American Journal of Public Health, 88,* 603–609.

Pizzo, B., Coyle, M., Seiverling, L., & Williams, K. (2012). Plate A–Plate B: Use of sequential presentation in the treatment of food selectivity. *Behavioral Interventions, 27,* 175–184.

Pizzo, B., Williams, K. E., Paul, C., & Riegel, K. (2009). Jump start exit criterion: Exploring a new model of service delivery for the treatment of childhood feeding problems. *Behavioral Interventions, 24,* 195–203.

Resnicow, K., Cohn, L., Reinhardt, J., Cross, D., Futterman, R., Kirschner, E., Wynder, E. L., & Allegrante, J. P. (1992). A three-year evaluation of the Know Your Body program in inner-city schoolchildren. *Health Education Quarterly, 19,* 463–480.

Reynolds, K. D., Franklin, F. A., Binkley, D., Raczynski, J. M., Harrington, K. F., Kirk, K. A., & Person, S. (2000). Increasing the fruit and vegetable consumption of fourth-graders: Results from the High-5 project. *Preventive Medicine, 30,* 309–319.

Rhoe, K. E., Lumeng, J. C., Appugliese, D. P., Kaciroti, N., & Bradley, R. H. (2006). Parent feeding styles and overweight status in first grade. *Pediatrics, 117,* 2047–2054.

Robinson, T. N. (1999). Behavioural treatment of childhood and adolescent obesity. *International Journal of Obesity and Related Metabolic Disorders, 23,* S52–S57.

Roe, L. S., Meengs, J. S., & Rolls, B. J. (2012). Salad and satiety: The effect of timing of salad consumption on meal energy intake. *Appetite, 58,* 242–248.

Rolls, B. J., Roe, L. S., & Meengs, J. S. (2004). Salad and satiety: Energy density and portion size of a first-course salad affect energy intake at lunch. *Journal of the American Dietetic Association, 104,* 1570–1576.

Rolls, B. J., Rolls, E. T., Rowe, E. A., & Sweeney, K. (1981). Sensory specific satiety in man. *Physiology and Behavior, 27,* 137–142.

Roseman, M. G., Riddell, M. C., & Haynes, J. N. (2010). A content analysis of kindergarten–12th grade school-based nutrition interventions: Taking advantage of past learning. *Journal of Nutrition Education and Behavior, 43,* 2–18.

Rozin, P. (1986). One-trial acquired likes and dislikes in humans: Disgust as a US, food predominance, and negative learning predominance. *Learning and Motivation, 17,* 180–189.

Rozin, P., Fischler, C., Shields, C., & Masson, E. (2006). Attitudes towards large numbers of choices in the food domain: A cross-cultural study of five countries in Europe and the USA. *Appetite, 46,* 304–308.

Sanders, M. R., Patel, R. K., LeGrice, B., & Shepard, R. W. (1993). Children with persistent feeding difficulties: An observational analysis of the feeding interactions of problem and non-problem eaters. *Health Psychology, 12,* 64–73.

Savage, J. S., Fisher, J. O., & Birch, L. L. (2007). Parental influence on eating behavior: Conception to adolescence. *Journal of Law and Medical Ethics, 35,* 22–34.

Schreck, K. A., Williams, K. E., & Smith, A. F. (2004). A comparison of eating behaviors between children with and without autism. *Journal of Autism and Developmental Disorders, 34,* 433–438.

Schwimmer, J. B., Burwinkle, T. M., & Varni, J. W. (2003). Health-related quality of life of severely obese children and adolescents. *Journal of the American Medical Association, 289,* 1813–1819.

Seiverling, L., Kokitus, A., & Williams, K. (2012). A clinical demonstration of a treatment package for food selectivity. *Behavior Analyst Today, 13,* 11–16.

Seiverling, L., Williams, K. E., & Hendy, H. M. (2011). The Screening Tool of Feeding Problems applied to children (the STEP–CHILD): Psychometric characteristics and associations with child and parent variables. *Research in Developmental Disabilities, 32,* 1122–1129.

Skinner, J. D., Carruth, B. R., Bounds, B., & Ziegler, P. J. (2002). Children's food preferences: A longitudinal analysis. *Journal of the American Dietetic Association, 102,* 1638–1647.

Spruijt-Metz, D., Lindquist, C. H., Birch, L. L., Fisher, J. O., & Goran, M. I. (2002). Relation between mothers' child-feeding practices and children's adiposity. *American Journal of Clinical Nutrition, 75,* 581–586.

Stark, L. J., Collins, F. L., Osnes, P. C., & Stokes, T. F. (1986). Using reinforcement and cueing to increase healthy snack food choices in preschoolers. *Journal of Applied Behavior Analysis, 19,* 367–379.

Story, M., Mays, R. W., Bishop, D. B., Perry, C. L., Taylor, G., Smyth, M., & Gray, C. (2000). 5-a-Day Power Plus: Process evaluation of a multicomponent elementary school program to increase fruit and vegetable consumption. *Health Education and Behavior, 27,* 187–200.

Sullivan, S. A., & Birch, L. L. (1990). Pass the sugar, pass the salt. *Developmental Psychology, 26,* 546–551.

Sullivan, S. A., & Birch, L. L. (1994). Infant dietary experience and acceptance of solid foods. *Pediatrics, 93,* 271–277.

Timimi, S., Douglas, J., & Tsiftssopoulou, K. (1997). Selective eaters: A retrospective case note study. *Child Care, Health and Development, 23,* 265–278.

Trost, S. G., Kerr, L. M., Ward, D. S., & Pate, R. R. (2001). Physical activity and determinants of physical activity in obese and non-obese children. *International Journal of Obesity and Related Metabolic Disorders, 25,* 822–829.

Turnbull, I. D., Heaslip, S., & McLeod, H. A. (2000). Preschool children's attitudes to fat and normal male and female stimulus figures. *International Journal of Obesity and Related Metabolic Disorders, 24,* 1705–1706.

Ventura, A. K., & Birch, L. L. (2008). Does parenting affect children's eating and weight status? *International Journal of Behavioral Nutrition and Physical Activity, 5,* 15. doi: 10.1186/1479–5868-5-15

Wang, Y., & Beydown, M. A. (2007). The obesity epidemic in the United States: Gender, age, socioeconomic, racial/ethnic, and geographic characteristics: A systematic review and meta-regression analysis. *Epidemiological Reviews, 29,* 6–28.

Wardle, J., & Carnell, S. (2006). Parental feeding practices and children's weight. *Acta Paediatrica, 96,* 5–11.

Wardle, J., Cooke, L., Gibson, E. L., Sapochnik, M., Sheilham, A., & Lawson, M. (2003). Increasing children's acceptance of vegetables: A randomized trial of parent-led exposure. *Appetite, 40,* 155–162.

Wardle, J., Guthrie, C. A., Sanderson, S., & Rapoport, L. (2001). Development of the Children's Eating Behavior Questionnaire. *Journal of Child Psychology and Psychiatry, 42,* 963–970.

Webber, L., Cooke, L., Hill, C., & Wardle, J. (2010). Child apidosity and maternal feeding practices: A longitudinal analysis. *American Journal of Clinical Nutrition, 92,* 1423–1442.

Williams, C. L., Gulli, M. T., & Deckelbaum, R. J. (2001). Prevention and treatment of childhood obesity. *Current Atherosclerosis Reports, 3,* 486–497.

Williams, K. E., Field, D. G., & Seiverling, L. (2010). Food refusal in children: A review of the literature. *Research in Developmental Disabilities, 31,* 625–633.

Williams, K. E., Gibbons, B., & Schreck, K. (2005) Comparing selective eaters with and without developmental disabilities. *Journal of Developmental and Physical Disabilities, 17,* 299–309.

Williams, K. E., Hendy, H. M., & Knecht, S. (2008). Parent feeding practices and child variables associated with childhood feeding problems. *Journal of Developmental and Physical Disabilities, 20,* 231–242.

Williams, K. E., Hendy, H. M., Seiverling, L., & Can, S. H. (2011). Validation of the Parent Mealtime Action Scale (PMAS) when applied to children referred to a hospital-based feeding clinic. *Appetite, 56,* 553–557.

Williams, K. E., Paul, C., Pizzo, B., & Riegel, K. (2008). Practice does make perfect: A longitudinal look at repeated taste exposure. *Appetite, 51,* 739–742.

Williams, K. E., & Seiverling, L. (2010). Eating problems in children in autism spectrum disorders. *Topics in Clinical Nutrition, 25,* 27–37.

Woo, K. S., Ping, C., Yu, C. W., Sung, R. Y. T., Quio, M., Leung, S. S. F., Lam, C. W. K., Metreweli, C., & Celermajar, D. D. (2004). Effects of diet and exercise on obesity-related vascular dysfunction in children. *Circulation, 109,* 1981–1986.

ACKNOWLEDGMENTS

We thank the children, parents, and school staff of Schuylkill Haven Area Elementary Center and Blue Mountain East Elementary School for their participation in the development of the Kid's Choice Program (KCP). We also thank Penn State University for the grants it provided in support of research to document KCP effectiveness. We are grateful to teams of undergraduate student-researchers from Penn State, Schuylkill Campus, who completed lunch and recess observations during KCP applications, conducted child interviews, and prepared questionnaire packets for parents and school staff. We appreciate the review of early drafts of the KCP guide provided by Eileen Smith, and translations of our Parent Mealtime Action Scale (PMAS) provided by Farideh Bowman, S. Hakan Can, Kyong-Mee Chung, Hartmut Heep, Maria Luiza Petty, Sunbul Rai, Mohammad Rezaei, Stephanie Unger, and Ping Wang. We thank Elsevier Publishing Company for permission to use our published figures documenting KCP effects on children's healthy behaviors and weight status. Finally, we are grateful to the Can family (Hakan, Hatice, Gunesh), the Godfrey family (Luke, Carinn, Ashlyn), the Hoppman family (Rick, Tabitha, Megan), and the Wheeler family (Ralph, Wendy, Lainie), and to John Hendy for providing photographs to illustrate important components of the Kid's Choice Program.

ABOUT THE AUTHORS

Dr. Helen Hendy is a professor of psychology at Penn State University, Schuylkill Campus. She received a Ph.D. in psychology from the University of California, Riverside, with her education and research funded by the National Science Foundation, the National Institute of Mental Health, and the Children's Miracle Network. After working with the legendary primatologist Jane Goodall to study social development of wild baboons in Africa, Dr. Hendy changed to an applied research specialization on school programs and parent actions associated with children's healthy diet and weight. She has produced more than fifteen publications on children's feeding behavior and more than thirty conference presentations for researchers, teachers, and parents. For this work, Dr. Hendy received two Citation Awards for Research Excellence from the Society of Behavioral Medicine. She resides in eastern Pennsylvania where she lifts weights, grows tomatoes, and makes treasure hunts for her nieces and nephews.

Dr. Keith Williams is the director of the feeding program at the Penn State Hershey Medical Center and professor of pediatrics at the Penn State College of Medicine. He has worked at the feeding program since its inception in 1997. During these years, the feeding program has treated children from 26 states and five countries outside the United States. Dr. Williams conducts workshops and training on the behavioral treatment of childhood feeding problems, both nationally and internationally. He has authored more than forty publications related to child feeding problems, including a recent book coauthored with Dr. Richard Foxx, *Treating Eating Problems of Children with Autism Spectrum Disorders and Developmental Disabilities*. Dr. Williams resides in central Pennsylvania with his wife, Sherri, and his two sons.

Mr. Thomas Camise received an M.Ed. in educational administration and an M.Ed. in elementary education with a concentration in special education from Lehigh University. He was director of special education and elementary principal for Schuylkill Haven Area School District, Pennsylvania. He also held positions in the Schuylkill County Intermediate Unit, including principal of special education classes, and special education teacher at both elementary and secondary levels. After 38 years in the field of education, Mr. Camise retired, although he currently serves as interim principal for a private school in Pennsylvania. His research focus is devoted to school-based child obesity prevention, with seven publications and eight conference presentations. Mr. Camise has been married for 37 years and has one son.

Made in the USA
San Bernardino, CA
08 March 2016